VEGAN
Breakfast and Brunch Recipes

Just In 30 Minutes

Copyright @ 2020 by Cookmaster's Kitchen.

All rights reserved worldwide.

No part of this publications may be reproduced, distributed, or transmitted in any form or by any means, including photocopying, recording, other electronic, or mechanical methods without writing permission from the publisher, except for the inclusion of brief quotations in a review.

Warning Disclaimer:

The purpose of this book is to educate and entertain. The author or publisher does not guarantee that anyone following the techniques, suggestions, ideas, or strategies will become successful. The author and publisher shall have neither liability or responsibility to anyone with respect to any loss or damage caused, or alleged to be caused, directly or indirectly by the information contained in this book.

ISBN: 9798634961675

A Vegan Cookbook with 100+ Easy and Tasty Recipes!

Start the day with kitchen-approved recipes for vegan pancakes, eggless crepes, tofu scramble, and more.

WHAT'S INSIDE

Vegan Waffles ------------------------- 6
Samoan Panikeke ---------------------- 7
Cranberry-Orange Spiced Oatmeal ----- 8
Vegan Pancakes ----------------------- 9
Authentic Potato Pancakes ------------ 10
Almond Berry Smoothie --------------- 11
Whole Wheat Vegan Drop Biscuits ---- 12
Peanut Butter and Maple Oatmeal ---- 13
Mangu -------------------------------- 14
Vegan Granola ----------------------- 15
Delicious Oat Bran Cereal ------------ 16
Amazing Tofu Scramble --------------- 17
Simple Fry Bread --------------------- 18
Steel-Cut Oats and Quinoa Breakfast - 19
Coconut Chocolate Chip Waffles ----- 20
Toasted Quinoa Granola -------------- 21
Garbanzo-Oat Pancakes -------------- 22
Vegan French Toast ------------------ 23
A+ Vegan Pancakes ------------------ 24
Chocolate-Hazelnut Marble Cake ----- 25
Oatmeal Energy Bars ----------------- 26
Two-Ingredient Banana Pancakes ----- 27
Pumpkin Apple Pie Smoothie --------- 28
Easy Vegan French Toast ------------ 29
Fluffy Vegan Pumpkin Pancakes ------ 30

Hearty Pumpkin Spice Oatmeal ------- 31
Warm Cinnamon Raisin Quinoa ------ 32
Light and Fluffy Vegan Waffles ------ 33
Vegan Vanilla Nut Oatmeal ----------- 34
Nut and Date Millet Porridge --------- 35
Vegan Chocolate Banana Oatmeal ---- 36
Chocolate Banana Oatmeal ----------- 37
Tempeh Breakfast Sausage Patties ---- 38
Lemon Poppy Seed Scones ----------- 39
Vegan Strawberry Oatmeal ----------- 40
Vegan Lemon Poppy Scones ---------- 41
Vegan Apple Carrot Muffins ---------- 42
Vegan Crepes ------------------------ 43
Mango Craze Juice Blend ------------ 44
Country Style Fried Potatoes --------- 45
Kale and Banana Smoothie ----------- 46
Muesli ------------------------------- 47
Avocado Toast (Vegan) --------------- 48
Rice and Raisin Breakfast Pudding ---- 49
Fava Bean Breakfast Spread ---------- 50
Quinoa Porridge --------------------- 51
Momma's Potatoes ------------------- 52
Whole Wheat Drop Biscuits ---------- 53
Cornmeal Mush ---------------------- 54
Oatmeal Chocolate Chip Pancakes ---- 55

WHAT'S INSIDE

- Blueberry Cornmeal Pancakes — 56
- Easy Vegan Whole Grain Pancakes — 57
- Eggless Crepes — 58
- Ultimate Tofu Breakfast — 59
- World's Best Vegan Pancakes — 60
- Refreshing Banana Drink — 61
- Blueberry Smoothie Bowl — 62
- Berry Good Smoothie II — 63
- Flax Seed Smoothie — 64
- Super food Chocolate Pudding — 65
- Raw Chia 'Porridge' — 66
- Berry Coconut Smoothie — 67
- Fasoulia — 68
- Matcha Coconut Smoothie — 69
- Akki Rotti — 70
- Anna's Scrambled Tofu — 71
- Fluffy Vegan Pancakes — 72
- Sunflower Banana Oatmeal — 73
- Orange Juice Goji Berries Smoothie — 74
- Strawberry Banana Smoothie — 75
- Strawberry-Banana Oatmeal — 76
- Orange Pancakes — 77
- Green Smoothie Bowl — 78
- Vegan Smoothie Bowl — 79
- Chia Ginger Smoothie — 80
- Orange Chia Smoothie — 81
- Banana Chocolate Smoothie — 82
- Acai Smoothie Bowl — 83
- Raw Mango Monster Smoothie — 84
- Vegan Morning Smoothie — 85
- Pina Colada Smoothie (Vegan) — 86
- Zucchini Smoothie — 87
- Fluffy Vegan Pumpkin Pancakes — 88
- Oatmeal-Banana Pancakes — 89
- Apple-Rosemary Steel-Cut Oats — 90
- Blueberry Mint Smoothie — 91
- Vegan Chocolate Smoothie — 92
- Whole Wheat Apple Pancakes — 93
- Chocolate Chip Vegan Bars — 94
- Kale Avocado Smoothie — 95
- Hearty Pumpkin Spice Oatmeal — 96
- Hearty Multigrain Seeded Bread — 97
- Avocado Smoothie — 98
- Detox Smoothie — 99
- Chia Pineapple Smoothie — 100
- Cucumber Pear Smoothie — 101
- Smoothie Bowl — 102
- Dreamy Cashew Butter Smoothie — 103
- Light and Fluffy Vegan Waffles — 104
- Quick Vegan Breakfast Bowl — 105
- Vegan Hazelnut Spread — 106

(RECIPE - 01)

VEGAN WAFFLES

These waffles are so yummy it feels sinful eating them. You can use rice milk instead of soy.

Prep Time:	Cooking Time:	Servings:
10 mins	30 mins	4

Ingredients

- 6 tablespoons water.
- 2 tablespoons flax seed meal.
- 1 cup rolled oats.
- 1 3/4 cups soy milk.
- 1/2 cup all-purpose flour.
- 1/2 cup whole wheat flour.
- 2 tablespoons canola oil.
- 4 teaspoons baking powder.
- 1 teaspoon vanilla extract.
- 1 tablespoon agave nectar.
- 1/2 teaspoon salt.

Directions:

01. Preheat a waffle iron according to manufacturer's instructions.

02. Stir water and flax seed meal together in a bowl.

03. Blend oats in a blender into a flour-like consistency. Add flax seed mixture, soy milk, all-purpose flour, whole wheat flour, canola oil, baking powder, vanilla extract, agave nectar, and salt to oats; blend until batter is just mixed.

04. Ladle 1/2 cup batter into preheated waffle iron. Cook the waffles according to manufacturer's instructions until golden and crisp, about 5 minutes.

(RECIPE - 02)

SAMOAN PANIKEKE

Per Serving: **337** calories; **11.4 g** fat; **54.9 g** carbohydrates; **4 g** protein; **0 mg** cholesterol; **83 mg** sodium.

Prep Time:	Cooking Time:	Servings:
10 mins	30 mins	12

Ingredients

- 3 1/2 cups all-purpose flour
- 1 1/3 cups white sugar
- 2 teaspoons baking powder
- 2 very ripe bananas, mashed
- 1 tablespoon vanilla extract
- 1 1/2 cups water
- 6 cups vegetable oil for frying

Directions:

01. Combine the flour, sugar, and baking powder in a bowl until thoroughly mixed, and stir in the bananas, vanilla extract, and water to make a smooth, sticky dough.

02. Heat oil in a deep-fryer or large saucepan to 350 degrees F (175 degrees C). The oil should be deep enough to completely cover the panikekes while frying, or at last 3 inches deep.

03. Scoop up a scant 1/4 cup of batter with a large spoon, and use another spoon to push it off into the oil. Fry in small batches of 4 or 5 until they float to the top and turn golden brown, about 3 minutes, then flip them to fry the other side. Remove from the fryer and let drain on paper towels.

(RECIPE - 03)

CRANBERRY-ORANGE SPICED OATMEAL

This is a wonderful microwave recipe for every morning! It's made with no added sugar, and plenty of oats and cinnamon for a warm, tasty breakfast.

Prep Time:	Cooking Time:	Servings:
5 mins	2 mins	1

Ingredients

- 3/4 cup old-fashioned rolled oats.
- 1/2 teaspoon ground cinnamon, or to taste.
- 1/4 cup dried cranberries.
- 1/2 cup frozen blueberries.
- 1/4 teaspoon ground turmeric (optional).
- 1 pinch ground ginger (optional).
- 1 cup water.
- 1/4 cup orange juice, or as needed.

Directions:

Place the rolled oats, cinnamon, cranberries, and blueberries in a microwave safe bowl. Add the turmeric and ginger, if desired. Pour in the water, and stir to mix ingredients. Cook on High until water is absorbed, about 2 minutes. Stir in orange juice to desired consistency.

(RECIPE - 04)

VEGAN PANCAKES

This vegan pancake recipe is the best of the vegan lot. The secret that these pancakes are not soggy like the other vegans ones is that it uses custard powder. This ensures the pancakes are cakelike and taste and look exactly like non-vegan pancakes. Mix fruit into the batter if you like. Serve hot with syrup or jam.

Prep Time:	Cooking Time:	Servings:
2 mins	20 mins	4

Ingredients

- 4 cups self-rising flour.
- 1 tablespoon white sugar.
- 1 tablespoon custard powder.
- 2 cups soy milk.

Directions:

01. In a large bowl, stir together the flour, sugar and custard powder. Mix in the soy milk with a whisk so there are no lumps.

02. Heat a griddle over medium heat, and coat with nonstick cooking spray. Spoon batter onto the surface, and cook until bubbles begin to form on the surface. Flip with a spatula and cook on the other side until golden.

(RECIPE - 05)

AUTHENTIC POTATO PANCAKES

An authentic European recipe for potato pancakes straight from Grandma!

Prep Time:	Cooking Time:	Servings:
30 mins	20 mins	10

Ingredients

- 10 russet potatoes, peeled and shredded.
- 1 carrot, peeled and shredded.
- 1 onion, finely diced.
- 5 cloves garlic, crushed.
- 1 tablespoon chopped flat leaf parsley.
- 1 tablespoon chopped fresh dill.
- 2 tablespoons fresh lemon juice.
- 1/4 cup olive oil.
- 2 tablespoons all-purpose flour.
- 2 cups dry bread crumbs.
- salt and pepper to taste.
- olive oil for frying, as needed.

Directions:

01. Mix potatoes, carrot, onion, garlic, parsley, and dill in a large bowl. Stir in lemon juice, 1/4 cup of olive oil, flour, bread crumbs, salt, and pepper. Knead just until mixture holds together.

02. Heat the remaining 1/4 cup olive oil in a skillet over medium heat. Working in batches, drop spoonfuls of potato mixture in hot oil. Cook approximately 4 minutes per side, or until golden brown. Serve hot.

(RECIPE - 06)

ALMOND BERRY SMOOTHIE

Almond milk and almond butter are the star ingredients in this berry smoothie for a nutritious, on-the-go meal that is vegan and paleo-friendly.

Prep Time:	Cooking Time	Servings:
10 mins	10 mins	1

Ingredients

- 1 cup frozen blueberries.
- 1 banana.
- 1/2 cup almond milk.
- 1 tablespoon almond butter.
- water as needed.

Directions:

Combine blueberries, banana, almond milk, and almond butter in a blender; blend until smooth, adding water for a thinner smoothie.

Nutrition Facts

Per Serving: **321** calories; **11.7 g** fat; **55.6 g** carbohydrates; **5.3 g** protein; **0 mg** cholesterol; **162 mg** sodium.

(RECIPE - 07)

WHOLE WHEAT VEGAN DROP BISCUITS

These vegan biscuits are quick, easy, and fluffy. They use all whole wheat flour.

Prep Time:	Cooking Time	Servings:
10 mins	10 mins	10

Ingredients

- 2 cups whole wheat flour.
- 4 teaspoons baking powder.
- 1 teaspoon salt.
- 2 tablespoons vegan butter.
- 2 tablespoons coconut oil.
- 1 cup almond milk.

Directions:

01. Preheat an oven to 450 degrees F (230 degrees C).

02. Mix flour, baking powder, and salt together in a bowl. Cut vegan butter and coconut oil into flour mixture using a fork until crumbly; stir in almond milk until just combined. Drop batter onto an ungreased baking sheet.

03. Bake in the preheated oven until biscuits are soft and lightly browned, 10 to 12 minutes

(RECIPE - 08)

PEANUT BUTTER AND MAPLE OATMEAL

This is a quick and tasty oatmeal recipe that I've really enjoyed. Even my daughter who doesn't like oatmeal will eat this right up!

Prep Time:	Cooking Time	Servings:
10 mins	5 mins	1

Ingredients

- 3/4 cup water.
- 1/4 cup steel-cut oats (such as Trader Joe's(R) Quick Cook Oats).
- 1 tablespoon natural peanut butter (such as Whole Foods 365 Organic Everyday Value(R)).
- 1 tablespoon maple syrup.
- 1/2 teaspoon brown sugar.

Directions:

01. Bring water to a boil in a saucepan, stir steel cut oats into water, and reduce heat to medium-low. Cover and cook until oats are tender, 5 to 7 minutes, stirring occasionally. Remove from heat and let stand 1 minute.

02. Stir peanut butter, maple syrup, and brown sugar into oats.

(RECIPE - 09)

MANGU

A Dominican favorite usually eaten in the morning.

Per Serving: 210 calories; **9.5 g** fat; **33.3 g** carbohydrates; **1.9 g** protein; **0 mg** cholesterol; **1756 mg** sodium.

Prep Time:	Cooking Time	Servings:
15 mins	25 mins	6

Ingredients

- 3 green plantains.
- 1 quart water.
- 1/4 cup olive oil.
- 1 cup sliced white onion.
- 1 1/2 tablespoons salt.
- 1 cup sliced Anaheim peppers.

Directions:

01. Place the plantains and water in a saucepan. Bring to a boil, and cook 20 minutes, until plantains are tender but slightly firm. Drain, reserving 1 cup of the liquid. Cool plantains, and peel.

02. Heat the olive oil in a skillet over medium heat, and saute the onion until tender.

03. In a bowl, mash the plantains with the reserved liquid and salt. Transfer to a food processor, mix in the peppers, and puree. Serve the pureed plantain mixture topped with the onions.

(RECIPE - 10)

VEGAN GRANOLA

This is an awesome, addictive, one hundred percent vegan granola. We always have a batch of this on hand to sprinkle on soy yogurt or eat with soy or rice milk.

Prep Time:	Cooking Time	Servings:
10 mins	30 mins	10

Ingredients

- cooking spray.
- 3 cups rolled oats.
- 2/3 cup wheat germ.
- 1/2 cup slivered almonds.
- 1 pinch ground nutmeg.
- 1 1/2 teaspoons ground cinnamon.
- 1/2 cup apple juice.
- 1/2 cup molasses.
- 1 teaspoon vanilla extract.
- 1 cup dried mixed fruit.
- 1 cup quartered dried apricots.

Directions:

01. Preheat oven to 350 degrees F (175 degrees C). Prepare two cookie sheets with cooking spray.

02. In a large bowl, combine oats, wheat germ, almonds, cinnamon and nutmeg. In a separate bowl, mix apple juice, molasses and extract. Pour the wet ingredients into the dry ingredients, stirring to coat. Spread mixture onto baking sheets.

03. Bake for 30 minutes in preheated oven, stirring mixture every 10 to 15 minutes, or until granola has a golden brown color. Let cool. Stir in dried fruit. Store in an airtight container.

(RECIPE - 11)

DELICIOUS OAT BRAN CEREAL

This recipe for a quick, hot breakfast cereal is sweetened with sugar substitute and dried plums.

Prep Time:	Cooking Time	Servings:
5 mins	5 mins	1

Ingredients

- 1 cup water.
- 1/4 teaspoon ground cinnamon.
- 5 dried pitted prunes, chopped.
- 1 teaspoon sugar substitute (such as Splenda).
- 1/4 cup oat bran.

Directions:

Combine water, cinnamon, prunes, and sugar substitute in a saucepan over medium heat; bring to a boil; stir in the oat bran and boil for 2 minutes.

Per Serving: **160** calories; **1.9 g** fat; **42.4 g** carbohydrates; **5.2 g** protein; **0 mg** cholesterol; **10 mg** sodium.

(RECIPE - 12)

AMAZING TOFU SCRAMBLE

Per Serving: 202 calories; **12.8 g** total fat; **0 mg** cholesterol; **140 mg** sodium. **10.3 g** carbohydrates; **14.7 g** protein

Prep Time:	Cooking Time	Servings:
15 mins	10 mins	2

Ingredients

- 2 teaspoons vegetable oil.
- ½ cup diced onion.
- ¼ cup minced carrot.
- ¼ cup diced fresh shiitake mushrooms.
- 1 (12 ounce) package firm tofu, crumbled.
- ½ teaspoon ground turmeric.
- ¼ teaspoon ground cumin.
- ⅛ teaspoon sea salt, or to taste.
- freshly ground black pepper to taste (optional).

Directions:

01. Heat oil in a skillet over medium heat; saute onion until softened, about 2 minutes. Add carrot to onion and saute until slightly softened, about 2 more minutes. Add mushrooms to onion mixture and saute until mushrooms are slightly tender, about 2 more minutes.

02. Stir tofu, turmeric, cumin, salt, and pepper into onion mixture; saute until tofu is cooked through, about 2 more minutes.

(RECIPE - 13)

SIMPLE FRY BREAD

This fry bread is easy to make and can be served with any meal or as dessert with jams, honey or, my favorite, maple syrup

Prep Time:	Cooking Time	Servings:
5 mins	15 mins	3

Ingredients

- vegetable oil for frying.
- 2 cups all-purpose flour.
- 1 tablespoon baking powder.
- 1 teaspoon salt.
- 3/4 cup water.

Directions:

01. Heat oil in a large saucepan to 350 degrees F (175 degrees C). Oil should be at least one-inch deep.

02. Mix flour, baking powder, and salt together in a large bowl. Add water a little at a time until dough comes together into a ball and doesn't stick to your hands, about 5 minutes.

03. Tear off plum-sized pieces of dough and flatten into 1/2-inch disks.

04. Fry pieces of dough in the hot oil until brown on both sides, about 3 minutes. Drain on paper towels or napkins before serving.

(RECIPE - 14)

STEEL-CUT OATS AND QUINOA BREAKFAST

The best make-ahead breakfast! Full of fiber and protein will keep you full all morning. Keeps in the fridge for up to a week.

Prep Time:	Cooking Time	Servings:
5 mins	20 mins	4

Ingredients

- 3 cups water.
- 1/2 cup quinoa.
- 1/2 cup steel-cut oats.
- 2 tablespoons almond meal.
- 2 tablespoons flaxseed meal.
- 1 tablespoon ground cinnamon.

Directions:

01. Bring water to a boil in a saucepan; add quinoa and oats. Simmer, stirring frequently, until water is absorbed and quinoa is tender, 15 to 20 minutes.

02. Stir almond meal and flaxseed meal into quinoa mixture; pour into a glass container and top with cinnamon. Let cool, about 15 minutes. Transfer to the refrigerator.

Per Serving: 191 calories; **4.7 g** fat; **30.6 g** carbohydrates; **7.6 g** protein; **0 mg** cholesterol; **8 mg** sodium.

(RECIPE - 15)

COCONUT CHOCOLATE CHIP WAFFLES

Looking for new waffle recipe? This one yields light, crispy waffles that your kids love. Choose your chocolate chips carefully, and your dish will be vegan as well!

Prep Time:	Cooking Time	Servings:
10 mins	15 mins	4

Ingredients

- 1 cup bread flour.
- 1 cup oat flour.
- 2 tablespoons white sugar.
- 1 tablespoon baking powder.
- 1/2 teaspoon ground cinnamon.
- 1/2 teaspoon salt.
- 1 2/3 cups unsweetened almond milk.
- 1/2 cup unsweetened applesauce.
- 1/3 cup coconut oil, melted.
- 1/2 cup chocolate chips.

Directions:

01. Preheat a waffle iron according to manufacturer's instructions.

02. Whisk bread flour, oat flour, sugar, baking powder, cinnamon, and salt together in a bowl. Mix almond milk, applesauce, and coconut oil together in a separate bowl; stir into flour mixture until batter is just combined. Fold chocolate chips into batter; let stand for 5 minutes.

03. Scoop 1/4 to 1/2 cup batter into preheated waffle iron; cook according to manufacturer's instructions, about 4 minutes per waffle.

(RECIPE - 16)

TOASTED QUINOA GRANOLA

Quick and easy. Sprinkle a few tablespoons of this nutty-tasting granola on yogurt. Quinoa is high in protein.

Prep Time:	Cooking Time	Servings:
15 mins	15 mins	10

Ingredients

- 1 cup quinoa.
- 1 tablespoon pure maple syrup.
- 1 tablespoon olive oil.
- 1 teaspoon ground cinnamon.
- 1/4 cup flax seed.

Directions:

01. Preheat oven to 350 degrees F (175 degrees C). Spray a baking sheet with cooking spray.

02. Rinse and thoroughly drain the quinoa. In a large bowl, stir together the maple syrup, olive oil, and cinnamon; mix in the quinoa and flax seed until the grains are thoroughly coated. Spread the mixture out as thinly as possible on the prepared baking sheet.

03. Toast the granola in the preheated oven until lightly golden brown, about 15 minutes, stirring every 5 minutes. Let cool completely before storing in an air-tight container.

(RECIPE - 17)

GARBANZO-OAT PANCAKES

Beans and grains combined make a nice combination. This recipe was developed for those on a wheat sensitive diet who can have gluten. It's great for people who need to be dairy and egg free. These do not form bubbles on the first side like 'normal' wheat pancakes. They do not brown like regular pancakes, either.

Prep Time:	Cooking Time	Servings:
5 mins	15 mins	4

Ingredients

- 1/2 cup garbanzo bean flour.
- 3/4 cup rolled oats.
- 1/4 cup yellow cornmeal.
- 1/2 teaspoon ground cinnamon.
- 1 teaspoon baking powder.
- 1 cup water.

Directions:

01. Stir the garbanzo bean flour, oats, cornmeal, cinnamon, and baking powder together in a mixing bowl until evenly blended. Stir in the water until only small lumps remain.

02. Heat a lightly oiled griddle over medium-high heat until a drop of water skitters across the surface. Drop batter by large spoonfuls onto the griddle, and cook until the edges are dry. Flip, and cook until browned on the other side, about 3 minutes per side. Repeat with remaining batter.

(RECIPE - 18)

VEGAN FRENCH TOAST

A delicious recipe for vegan French toast. Spice it up with 1/3 teaspoon nutmeg, cloves, or 1/4 teaspoon pumpkin pie spice. Add a mashed banana or a few tablespoons of applesauce to the mix for added sweetness and flavor. Add fresh berries or crushed nuts to the mix if you wish for even more variety. Of course, finish it off with a drizzle of maple syrup for an amazing dairy-free, egg-free, vegan breakfast.

Prep Time:	Cooking Time	Servings:
10 mins	10 mins	2

Ingredients

- 1 cup soy milk.
- 2 tablespoons all-purpose flour.
- 1 tablespoon nutritional yeast.
- 1 teaspoon raw sugar.
- 1 teaspoon vanilla extract.
- 1/3 teaspoon ground cinnamon.
- 4 slices bread.

Directions:

01. Whisk soy milk, flour, nutritional yeast, sugar, vanilla extract, and cinnamon together in a bowl; transfer to a rimmed plate or shallow dish. Dip both sides of each bread slice in soy milk mixture.

02. Heat a lightly oiled skillet over medium-low heat. Cook each slice of bread until golden brown, 3 to 4 minutes per side.

Per Serving: 254 calories; 4 g fat; 42.7 g carbohydrates; 10.6 g protein; 0 mg cholesterol; 405 mg sodium.

(RECIPE - 19)

A+ VEGAN PANCAKES

Packed with all you need in a breakfast. You can freeze them and reheat in a toaster. YUM!

Prep Time:	Cooking Time	Servings:
10 mins	10 mins	7

Ingredients

- 2 cups spelt flour.
- 2 cups oat flour.
- 2 tablespoons baking powder.
- 1/4 cup ground flaxseed meal.
- 1/2 teaspoon salt.
- 3 1/2 cups low-fat vanilla soy milk.
- 1/4 cup applesauce.
- 2 tablespoons agave nectar.
- 1 1/2 tablespoons vanilla extract.
- 2 cups blueberries.

Directions:

01. Whisk spelt flour, oat flour, baking powder, flaxseed meal, and salt together in a large mixing bowl.

02. Stir soy milk, applesauce, agave nectar, and vanilla extract together in a separate bowl.

03. Form a well in the center of the flour mixture and pour soy milk mixture into the well. Stir until the ingredients are just moistened; set aside for 15 minutes.

04. Lightly oil and heat a griddle to medium heat.

05. Spoon batter onto hot griddle, sprinkle blueberries onto wet batter, and cook until bubbles form, 2 to 3 minutes. Flip and continue cooking until golden brown on both sides, about 3 minutes more.

(RECIPE - 20)

CHOCOLATE-HAZELNUT MARBLE CAKE SCONES

These easy scones with dark chocolate chips and a hint of hazelnut are perfect for brunch or a tea-time snack.

Prep Time:	Cooking Time	Servings:
15 mins	20 mins	8

Ingredients

- 2 cups all-purpose flour.
- 1/4 cup sugar.
- 1 1/2 teaspoons baking powder.
- 1/2 teaspoon salt.
- 1/2 teaspoon baking soda.
- 6 tablespoons vegan butter.
- 2/3 cup So Delicious(R) Dairy Free Hazelnut Coconut Milk Creamer.
- 1/3 cup dark chocolate chips.

Directions:

01. Preheat oven to 425 degrees F. Line a baking sheet with parchment paper. Sift together flour, sugar, baking powder, salt, and baking soda in large bowl. Add vegan butter and mix together with hands until mixture forms large, coarse crumbs the size of peas. Add chocolate chips and creamer, mix for a few more seconds until just moistened. Turn the dough onto a lightly floured work surface and press together gently until the dough clings together in a ball. Pat into a circle about 2-inches thick and 6 inches in diameter.

02. Let sit for 15 minutes at room temperature. Cut into 8 wedges. Sprinkle with remaining tablespoon of sugar.

03. Bake for 15-20 minutes or until golden on top. Allow to cool for a few minutes, before separating wedges.

(RECIPE - 21)
OATMEAL ENERGY BARS

These tasty vegan energy bars taste just like full-fat, non-vegan oatmeal cookies. Completely irresistible. They are great as breakfast bars with coffee, as an in-between meal snack to keep you going, or a healthy dessert! Once you try them, you will never bother with non-vegan oatmeal cookies again!

Prep Time:	Cooking Time	Servings:
15 mins	15 mins	24

Ingredients

- 1 ⅓ cups rolled oats.
- ½ cup all-purpose flour.
- ½ cup vegan semi-sweet chocolate chips.
- ½ cup ground unsalted cashews.
- 2 tablespoons shelled unsalted sunflower seeds.
- 1 tablespoon ground flax meal.
- 1 tablespoon wheat germ.
- ½ teaspoon ground cinnamon.
- ¼ teaspoon sea salt.
- ½ cup honey, warmed.
- ⅓ cup almond butter.
- ½ teaspoon vanilla extract.

Directions:

01. Preheat oven to 350 degrees F (175 degrees C). Line a 9x11-inch baking dish with aluminum foil.

02. Whisk oats, flour, chocolate chips, ground cashews, sunflower seeds, flax meal, wheat germ, cinnamon, and sea salt together in a large shallow bowl.

03. Stir warmed honey, almond butter, and vanilla extract together in a bowl until well-mixed. Pour honey mixture into oat mixture; stir until batter is well-combined. Turn batter out into prepared baking dish. Lay a sheet of waxed paper over batter and press firmly to evenly distribute in the baking dish. Remove and discard waxed paper.

04. Bake in the preheated oven until golden and fragrant, about 12 minutes. Pull aluminum foil from baking dish and cool bars in the aluminum foil for 10 minutes; remove and discard aluminum foil. Cut into bars.

(RECIPE - 22)

TWO-INGREDIENT BANANA PANCAKES

The quickest and easiest pancake recipe ever! Perfect use of those soft bananas.

Prep Time:	Cooking Time	Servings:
3 mins	2 mins	1

Ingredients

- 1 ripe banana.
- 1 egg.
- 1/2 teaspoon vanilla extract (optional).

Directions:

01. Mix banana and egg together in a bowl until no lumps remain. Add vanilla extract to the batter.

02. Heat a greased skillet or griddle over medium heat. Pour batter into the pan. Cook until bubbles appear, about 1 minute. Flip and cook until golden, about 1 minute more.

Per Serving: 78 calories; **5 g** fat; **0.7 g** carbohydrates; **6.3 g** protein; **186 mg** cholesterol; **70 mg** sodium.

(RECIPE - 23)

PUMPKIN APPLE PIE SMOOTHIE

This healthy, delicious vegan smoothie is perfect when you're craving fall flavors in the heat of the summer! Perfect for a low calorie breakfast or an energy-packed snack. Top with crushed graham crackers, pecans, granola, or whipped cream if desired.

Prep Time:	Cooking Time	Servings:
10 mins	5 mins	1

Ingredients

- 1 apple - peeled, cored, and chopped.
- 2 tablespoons water, or as needed.
- 2/3 cup unsweetened vanilla-flavored almond milk.
- 1/4 cup pumpkin puree.
- 1 1/2 teaspoons brown sugar, or to taste.
- 1/4 teaspoon pumpkin pie spice.
- 2/3 cup crushed ice cubes.

Directions:

01. Place apple in a plastic microwave-safe bowl; pour in enough water to cover 1/4-inch of the bottom of bowl. Partially cover bowl with a lid or paper towel. Microwave in 1 minute intervals until apple is softened, 2 to 3 minutes. Freeze apple in the same container with water until solid, 2 hours to overnight.

02. Blend frozen apple, almond milk, and pumpkin puree in a blender until smooth; add brown sugar and pumpkin pie spice. Blend until smooth. Add ice and blend until smooth.

(RECIPE - 24)

EASY VEGAN FRENCH TOAST

Try vegan French toast for dairy-free deliciousness! We use soy milk, but almond or other non-dairy milk might work. You could also add some nutritional yeast to the batter, if you like.

Prep Time:	Cooking Time	Servings:
5 mins	5 mins	2

Ingredients

- 1 1/2 cups soy milk.
- 2 tablespoons all-purpose flour.
- 1 teaspoon white sugar.
- 1 teaspoon ground cinnamon.
- 1 tablespoon vegetable oil.
- 4 slices bread, or more as needed.

Directions:

01. Whisk soy milk, flour, sugar, and cinnamon together in a bowl until well beaten. Pour into a pie pan or other wide, shallow dish.

02. Heat oil in a skillet over medium-high heat.

03. Dip each slice of bread into the soy milk mixture and place into the skillet. Cook until golden brown and crispy on both sides, 5 to 7 minutes.

Per Serving: **331** calories; **11.7 g** fat; **45.7 g** carbohydrates; **10.6 g** protein; **0 mg** cholesterol; **434 mg** sodium.

(RECIPE - 25)

FLUFFY VEGAN PUMPKIN PANCAKES

Pumpkin puree turns these vegan pancakes orange and adds flavor. Use whatever nondairy milk you prefer. Enjoy with toppings such as nuts or bananas and syrup!

Prep Time:	Cooking Time	Servings:
10 mins	10 mins	3

Ingredients

- 1 1/4 cups all-purpose flour.
- 2 teaspoons baking powder.
- 1 teaspoon pumpkin pie spice.
- 1/2 teaspoon salt.
- 1 cup soy milk.
- 1 tablespoon brown sugar.
- 3 tablespoons pumpkin puree.
- 1 teaspoon vanilla extract.
- 1 1/2 teaspoons vegetable oil.
- 1/3 cup water.

Directions:

01. Combine flour, baking powder, pumpkin pie spice, and salt in a bowl.

02. Stir milk, brown sugar, pumpkin puree, vanilla extract, oil, and water together in a second bowl; mix thoroughly. Make a well in the flour mixture, add milk mixture, and mix until evenly combined.

03. Heat a nonstick skillet over medium-high heat. Drop 1/4 cup pancake batter onto the hot skillet and cook until bubbles form and edges are dry, 3 to 5 minutes. Flip and cook until browned on the other side, 3 to 5 minutes. Repeat with remaining batter.

(RECIPE - 26)

HEARTY PUMPKIN SPICE OATMEAL

Delicious breakfast for fall.

Prep Time:	Cooking Time	Servings:
5 mins	13 mins	2

Ingredients

- 2 cups unsweetened almond milk.
- 1/2 cup pumpkin puree.
- 2 tablespoons maple syrup.
- 1 teaspoon vanilla extract.
- 1/4 teaspoon ground cinnamon.
- 1/4 teaspoon ground nutmeg.
- 1/4 teaspoon ground cloves.
- 1 cup old-fashioned oats.

Directions:

Combine almond milk, pumpkin puree, maple syrup, vanilla extract, cinnamon, nutmeg, and cloves in a saucepan over medium heat; bring to a boil. Add oatmeal and cook, stirring frequently, until chewy and tender, 8 to 10 minutes.

Cook's Note:
Instead of using 2 cups of almond milk, you can use 1 cup milk and 1 cup water.

Per Serving: 300 calories; **5.7 g** fat; **55.2 g** carbohydrates; **7.1 g** protein; **0 mg** cholesterol; **313 mg** sodium.

(RECIPE - 27)

WARM CINNAMON RAISIN QUINOA

When ready to eat, place a portion of the quinoa into a bowl, drizzle with maple syrup and top with chia seeds, raisins, and nut butter.

Prep Time:	Cooking Time	Servings:
10 mins	20 mins	4

Ingredients

- 2 cups almond milk.
- 1 cup quinoa.
- 1 teaspoon ground cinnamon.
- 5 vanilla beans.
- 1 cup raisins.
- 2 tablespoons chia seeds, or to taste.
- 2 tablespoons ground flax seeds, or to taste.

Directions:

01. Bring almond milk and quinoa to a boil in a saucepan. Add cinnamon and vanilla beans; reduce heat and simmer, stirring occasionally, until all liquid is absorbed, about 15 minutes. Remove vanilla beans from quinoa.

02. Spoon quinoa into bowls; top each with raisins, chia seeds, and ground flax seeds.

Per Serving: **419** calories; **6.7 g** fat; **84.6 g** carbohydrates; **9 g** protein; **0 mg** cholesterol; **88 mg** sodium.

(RECIPE - 28)

LIGHT AND FLUFFY VEGAN WAFFLES

Simple, vegan waffle recipe for a lazy weekend morning. Cooked waffles store well in the fridge or frozen and reheat in the toaster, if allowed to cool fully and kept separated between sheets of parchment paper.

Prep Time:	Cooking Time	Servings:
10 mins	30 mins	6

Ingredients

- 1/2 cup warm water.
- 2 tablespoons flaxseed meal.
- 2 cups all-purpose flour.
- 2 tablespoons baking powder.
- 1 tablespoon white sugar.
- 1/2 teaspoon salt.
- 1 3/4 cups almond milk.
- 1/4 cup vegetable oil.
- 1/4 cup applesauce.
- 1 teaspoon vanilla extract.

Directions:

01. Combine water and flaxseed meal in a medium-sized bowl. Set aside for 5 minutes.

02. Combine flour, baking powder, sugar, and salt in a large mixing bowl. Mix well.

03. Add almond milk, oil, applesauce, and vanilla extract to flaxseed mixture. Combine until smooth. Add to flour mixture and stir until just combined.

04. Preheat a waffle iron according to manufacturer's instructions.

05. Add 1/3 cup waffle batter to the preheated waffle iron and cook until waffle is golden brown and the iron stops steaming, about 5 minutes. Repeat with remaining batter.

(RECIPE - 29)

VEGAN VANILLA NUT OATMEAL

Enjoy this quick to make, delicious, vegan-friendly oatmeal. It's so versatile, it can serve as a breakfast, lunch, dinner, or a pre-/post-workout option.

Prep Time:	Cooking Time	Servings:
5 mins	10 mins	1

Ingredients

- 3/4 cup vanilla soy milk.
- 1/2 cup rolled oats.
- 2 teaspoons white sugar.
- 2 teaspoons chia seeds (optional).
- 2 teaspoons chopped almonds.
- 1 teaspoon vanilla bean powder.
- 1/4 teaspoon sea salt.
- 1/4 teaspoon ground cinnamon.

Directions:

Combine soy milk, oats, sugar, chia seeds, almonds, vanilla bean powder, salt, and cinnamon in a saucepan over medium heat. Cook and stir frequently until thickened to your preference, 5 to 7 minutes.

Cook's Notes:
You can use 1/2 teaspoon of vanilla extract in place of the vanilla bean powder. You can use coconut or maple sugar, if you prefer. Use any nuts of your choice.

Per Serving: 352 calories; **9.4 g** fat; **55.3 g** carbohydrates; **12.9 g** protein; **0 mg** cholesterol; **536 mg** sodium.

(RECIPE - 30)
NUT AND DATE MILLET PORRIDGE

This millet porridge with nuts and dates is vegan and gluten-free.

Prep Time:	Cooking Time	Servings:
10 mins	30 mins	2

Ingredients

- 1/2 cup hulled millet.
- 2 tablespoons slivered almonds.
- 2 tablespoons pepitas.
- 2 tablespoons shredded unsweetened coconut.
- 1 tablespoon flax seeds.
- 2 cups unsweetened almond milk, divided.
- 3 medjool dates, pitted and diced.
- 1/2 teaspoon ground cinnamon.
- 1/4 teaspoon ground nutmeg.

Directions:

01. Pulse millet in a blender or food processor until it resembles coarse ground coffee. Set aside.

02. Heat a nonstick saucepan over medium-high heat. Add almonds and toast until golden brown, stirring occasionally, about 2 minutes. Add pepitas and continue to stir and toast until golden brown, about 3 minutes. Stir in coconut and flax seeds and toast until golden, about 5 minutes more. Pour mixture into a bowl and set aside.

03. Pour ground millet into the same pan. Toast until fragrant, about 3 minutes. Pour in 1 1/2 cups almond milk, stirring to ensure there are no lumps. Bring to a boil; add dates. Reduce heat to medium and simmer, stirring occasionally.

04. Add 2 tablespoons of the toasted seed mixture to the porridge. Sprinkle in cinnamon and nutmeg. Stir well. Continue simmering until thickened, 6 to 10 minutes.

05. Pour porridge into two bowls. Divide remaining seed mixture and 1/2 cup almond milk between bowls and serve.

(RECIPE - 31)

VEGAN CHOCOLATE BANANA OATMEAL

A wholesome and yummy vegan chocolate oatmeal.

Prep Time:	Cooking Time	Servings:
5 Mins	10 mins	1

Ingredients

- 3/4 cup cashew milk.
- 1/4 cup quick-cooking oats.
- 1 teaspoon unsweetened cocoa powder.
- 1 pinch salt.
- 1 pinch ground cinnamon.
- 2 teaspoons maple syrup, or more to taste.
- 1 tablespoon vegan dark chocolate chips.
- 1/2 banana, sliced.

Directions:

01. Pour cashew milk into a saucepan and bring to a boil over medium-high heat. Add oats and reduce heat to a simmer. Stir in cocoa powder, salt, and cinnamon until well combined. Sweeten with maple syrup. Simmer for 5 minutes. Add chocolate chips, stir, and cook until oatmeal has desired consistency, 1 to 2 minutes more.

02. Pour oatmeal into a bowl and top with banana.

Cook's Note:
We have also used almond milk instead of cashew milk.

(RECIPE - 32)
REDUCED-CALORIE CHOCOLATE BANANA OATMEAL

Chocolate-banana oatmeal is a yummy treat.

Prep Time:	Cooking Time	Servings:
5 Mins	5 mins	1

Ingredients

- 2 tablespoons unsweetened cocoa powder.
- 1/8 teaspoon ground cinnamon.
- 1 packet zero-calorie sweetener.
- 1 pinch salt.
- 1/4 cup hot water.
- 1/4 cup cold water.
- 1/3 cup rolled oats.
- 1/2 banana, mashed.

Directions:

01. Pour cocoa powder into a microwave-safe bowl and stir in cinnamon, sweetener, and salt. Add hot water and stir thoroughly until cocoa powder has dissolved. Stir in cold water until well combined. Stir in oats and banana until mixed well.

02. Microwave for 2 minutes. Remove, stir, and allow oatmeal to cool and thicken.

Cook's Note:
You can also use a 25-calorie packet of diet hot cocoa mix instead of unsweetened cocoa powder.

(RECIPE - 33)

TEMPEH BREAKFAST SAUSAGE PATTIES

This is a great vegan, cholesterol-free alternative to pork breakfast sausage. It's very easy to make and can be made ahead for a quick weekday breakfast

Prep Time:	Cooking Time	Servings:
10 Mins	13 mins	11

Ingredients

- 1 (8 ounce) package tempeh, grated.
- 1/4 cup tamari.
- 3 cloves garlic, crushed, or more to taste.
- 2 1/2 teaspoons dried sage.
- 1 1/2 teaspoons smoked paprika.
- 1 teaspoon ground black pepper.
- 2 teaspoons red pepper flakes.
- 1/4 cup whole wheat flour.
- 1/2 teaspoon olive oil, or as needed.

Directions:

01. Combine tempeh, tamari, garlic, sage, paprika, black pepper, and red pepper flakes in a saucepan. Simmer, stirring tempeh frequently, until completely reduced, about 7 minutes.

02. Stir flour into tempeh mixture. Let cool in the saucepan until safe to handle, about 15 minutes. Shape into 2-inch patties.

03. Heat a skillet over medium heat and grease with olive oil. Pan-fry the patties until well-browned, about 3 minutes per side. Drain on paper towels.

(RECIPE - 34)
LEMON POPPY SEED SCONES

These are scrumptious little scones that will satisfy those with allergies or gluten free, dairy free, or vegan lifestyle.

Prep Time:	Cooking Time	Servings:
15 Mins	15 mins	8

Ingredients

- 9 tablespoons water.
- 3 tablespoons ground flax seeds.
- 1/4 cup maple syrup.
- 3 tablespoons coconut oil, melted.
- 1 lemon, zested and juiced.
- 1 teaspoon vanilla extract.
- 2/3 cup oat flour.
- 1/3 cup white rice flour.
- 1/4 cup brown rice flour.
- 2 tablespoons coconut flour.
- 1 tablespoon poppy seeds.
- 1 teaspoon baking soda.
- 1 teaspoon baking powder.
- 1/2 teaspoon xanthan gum.
- 1/4 teaspoon salt.

Directions:

01. Preheat oven to 350 degrees F (175 degrees C). Grease a baking sheet.

02. Whisk water and ground flax seeds together in a small bowl. Let stand until thickened, about 5 minutes. Mix in maple syrup, coconut oil, lemon zest, lemon juice, and vanilla extract.

03. Mix oat flour, white rice flour, brown rice flour, coconut flour, poppy seeds, baking soda, baking powder, xanthan gum, and salt together in a large bowl. Add maple syrup mixture; mix with a spatula until dough comes together in a ball.

04. Transfer ball of dough to a large sheet of waxed paper; press into a circle about 1 inch thick. Cut into 8 wedges. Pull wedges apart and carefully transfer to the prepared baking sheet.

05. Bake in the preheated oven until golden brown, 15 to 17 minutes. Cool on a wire rack.

(RECIPE - 35)

VEGAN STRAWBERRY OATMEAL BREAKFAST SMOOTHIE

This is a fast and filling vegan smoothie with a deep pink color and a rich, creamy texture.

Prep Time:	Ready Time	Servings:
10 Mins	10 mins	2

Ingredients

- 1 cup almond milk
- 1/2 cup rolled oats
- 14 frozen strawberries
- 1 banana, broken into chunks
- 1 1/2 teaspoons agave nectar (optional)
- 1/2 teaspoon vanilla extract (optional)

Directions:

Blend almond milk, oats, strawberries, banana, agave nectar, and vanilla extract in a blender until smooth.

Cook's Note:
Rice milk can be used in place of the almond milk. Two packets of stevia sweetener can replace the agave syrup, if preferred.

(RECIPE - 36)

VEGAN LEMON POPPY SCONES

Delicious lemon poppy scones that happen to be vegan. Note, this recipe can be changed up quite easily. And the proportions are pretty forgiving, too. Experiment with different sweeteners and flours if you like. These are very adaptable.

Prep Time:	Cooking Time	Servings:
10 Mins	15 mins	12

Ingredients

- 2 cups all-purpose flour
- 3/4 cup white sugar
- 4 teaspoons baking powder
- 1/2 teaspoon salt
- 3/4 cup vegan margarine
- 1 lemon, zested and juiced
- 2 tablespoons poppy seeds
- 1/2 cup soy milk
- 1/2 cup water

Directions:

01. Preheat the oven to 400 degrees F (200 degrees C). Grease a baking sheet.

02. Sift the flour, sugar, baking powder and salt into a large bowl. Cut in margarine until the mixture is the consistency of large grains of sand. I like to use my hands to rub the margarine into the flour. Stir in poppy seeds, lemon zest and lemon juice. Combine the soy milk and water, and gradually stir into the dry ingredients until the batter is moistened, but still thick like biscuit dough. You may not need all of the liquid.

03. Spoon 1/4 cup sized plops of batter onto the greased baking sheet so they are about 3 inches apart.

04. Bake for 10 to 15 minutes the preheated oven, until golden.

(RECIPE - 37)

VEGAN APPLE CARROT MUFFINS

Vegan egg substitute is a powder that you add water to, and can be bought at most grocery stores. It is fat free, vegan and has few calories per 'egg'. If you can't find it, use 6 eggs, but remember that the fat content will go way up.

Prep Time:	Cooking Time	Servings:
20 Mins	20 mins	12

Ingredients

- 1 cup brown sugar
- 1/2 cup white sugar
- 2 1/2 cups all-purpose flour
- 4 teaspoons baking soda
- 1 teaspoon baking powder
- 4 teaspoons ground cinnamon
- 2 teaspoons salt
- 2 cups finely grated carrots
- 2 large apples - peeled, cored and shredded
- 6 teaspoons egg replacer (dry)
- 1 1/4 cups applesauce
- 1/4 cup vegetable oil

Directions:

01. Preheat oven to 375 degrees F (190 degrees C). Grease muffin cups or line with paper muffin liners.

02. In a large bowl combine brown sugar, white sugar, flour, baking soda, baking powder, cinnamon and salt. Stir in carrot and apple; mix well.

03. In a small bowl whisk together egg substitute, applesauce and oil. Stir into dry ingredients.

04. Spoon batter into prepared pans.

05. Bake in preheated oven for 20 minutes. Let muffins cool in pan for 5 minutes before removing from pans to cool completely.

(RECIPE - 38)

VEGAN CREPES

This is the first recipe for crepes that we have ever been able to make right. We was psyched that we didn't have to use egg replacer because it is such a pain in the neck. So here you vegans go and enjoy but don't eat too many too fast like we did cause now we have a belly ache!!!!

Prep Time:	Cooking Time	Servings:
5 Mins	20 mins	4

Ingredients

- 1/2 cup soy milk.
- 1/2 cup water.
- 1/4 cup melted soy margarine.
- 1 tablespoon turbinado sugar.
- 2 tablespoons maple syrup.
- 1 cup unbleached all-purpose flour.
- 1/4 teaspoon salt.

Directions:

01. In a large mixing bowl, blend soy milk, water, 1/4 cup margarine, sugar, syrup, flour, and salt. Cover and chill the mixture for 2 hours.

02. Lightly grease a 5 to 6 inch skillet with some soy margarine. Heat the skillet until hot. Pour approximately 3 tablespoons batter into the skillet. Swirl to make the batter cover the skillet's bottom. Cook until golden, flip and cook on opposite side.

(RECIPE - 39)

MANGO CRAZE JUICE BLEND

A great smoothie for the true mango lover!

Prep Time:	Ready Time	Servings:
5 Mins	5 mins	4

Ingredients

- 3 cups diced mango.
- 1 1/2 cups chopped fresh or frozen peaches.
- 1/4 cup chopped orange segments.
- 1/4 cup chopped and pitted nectarine.
- 1/2 cup orange juice.
- 2 cups ice.

Directions:

Place mango, peaches, orange, nectarine, orange juice, and ice into a blender. Blend for 1 minute, or until smooth.

(RECIPE - 40)

COUNTRY STYLE FRIED POTATOES

These fried potatoes are the perfect companion for bacon and eggs. You may use oil instead of shortening if you wish.

Prep Time:	Cooking Time	Servings:
10 Mins	15 mins	6

Ingredients

- 1/3 cup shortening.
- 6 large potatoes, peeled and cubed.
- 1 teaspoon salt.
- 1 teaspoon salt.
- 1/2 teaspoon ground black pepper.
- 1/2 teaspoon garlic powder.
- 1/2 teaspoon paprika.

Directions:

In a large cast iron skillet, heat shortening over medium-high heat. Add potatoes and cook, stirring occasionally, until potatoes are golden brown. Season with salt, pepper, garlic powder and paprika. Serve hot.

(RECIPE - 41)

KALE AND BANANA SMOOTHIE

Nutrient-rich kale is hidden in this delicious banana smoothie... perfect for those of us who have a hard time getting our daily dose of veggies!

Prep Time:	Ready Time	Servings:
5 Mins	5 mins	1

Ingredients

- 1 banana.
- 2 cups chopped kale.
- 1/2 cup light unsweetened soy milk.
- 1 tablespoon flax seeds
- 1 teaspoon maple syrup

Directions:

Place the banana, kale, soy milk, flax seeds, and maple syrup into a blender. Cover, and puree until smooth. Serve over ice.

(RECIPE - 42)

MUESLI

This is a nutritious and delicious breakfast cereal. Use any type of dried fruit you desire! You can also use almonds in place of walnuts if you like. Wonderful when served in bowls with milk and fresh berries or sliced fresh fruit.

Prep Time:	Ready Time	Servings:
10 Mins	10 mins	16

Ingredients

- 4 1/2 cups rolled oats
- 1/2 cup toasted wheat germ
- 1/2 cup wheat bran
- 1/2 cup oat bran
- 1 cup raisins
- 1/2 cup chopped walnuts
- 1/4 cup packed brown sugar
- 1/4 cup raw sunflower seeds

Directions:

In a large mixing bowl combine oats, wheat germ, wheat bran, oat bran, dried fruit, nuts, sugar, and seeds. Mix well. Store muesli in an airtight container. It keeps for 2 months at room temperature.

(RECIPE - 43)

AVOCADO TOAST (VEGAN)

This is a delicious, healthy, hearty breakfast recipe. If you are not vegan, you can add fried eggs to your toast for a delicious vegetarian meal.

Prep Time:	Ready Time	Servings:
10 Mins	10 mins	4

Ingredients

- 4 slices whole-grain bread.
- 1 avocado, halved and pitted.
- 2 tablespoons chopped fresh parsley.
- 1 1/2 teaspoons extra-virgin olive oil.
- 1/2 lemon, juiced.
- 1/2 teaspoon salt.
- 1/2 teaspoon ground black pepper.
- 1/2 teaspoon onion powder.
- 1/2 teaspoon garlic powder.

Directions:

01. Toast bread in a toaster or toaster oven.

02. Scoop avocado into a bowl. Add parsley, olive oil, lemon juice, salt, pepper, onion powder, and garlic powder; mash together using a potato masher. Spread avocado mixture into each piece of toast.

(RECIPE - 44)

RICE AND RAISIN BREAKFAST PUDDING

A good use for leftover rice. Can be served hot or cold.

Prep Time:	Cooking Time	Servings:
5 Mins	10 mins	4

Ingredients

- 3 cups cooked brown rice.
- 1 cup soy milk.
- 1/2 cup raisins.
- 1/2 cup toasted and chopped almonds.
- 1/4 cup maple syrup.
- 1 teaspoon ground cinnamon.
- 1/2 teaspoon ground cardamom.

Directions:

Combine rice, soy milk, raisins, almonds, maple syrup, cinnamon, and cardamom in a saucepan; bring to a boil over medium-high heat. Reduce heat to low and simmer, stirring frequently to prevent scorching, until thickened, 5 to 8 minutes. Spoon into 4 bowls.

(RECIPE - 45)

FAVA BEAN BREAKFAST SPREAD

A deliciously seasoned fava bean, onion, and tomato dip recipe! Traditionally served with pita bread for breakfast in Egypt.

Prep Time:	Cooking Time	Servings:
10 Mins	10 mins	6

Ingredients

- 1 (15 ounce) can fava beans.
- 1 1/2 tablespoons olive oil.
- 1 large onion, chopped.
- 1 large tomato, diced.
- 1 teaspoon ground cumin.
- 1/4 cup chopped fresh parsley.
- 1/4 cup fresh lemon juice.
- salt and pepper to taste.
- ground red pepper, to taste.

Directions:

Pour the beans into a pot and bring to a boil. Mix them well and add onion, tomato, olive oil, cumin, parsley, lemon juice, salt, pepper, and red pepper. Bring the mixture back to a boil, then reduce the heat to medium. Let the mixture cook 5 minutes. Serve warm with grilled pita.

(RECIPE - 46)

QUINOA PORRIDGE

Here's a dairy and wheat free breakfast porridge thick, rich and delish for those cold mornings in the Andes. Those with nut allergies may wish to substitute soymilk or regular cow's milk for the almond. Adjust sugar to your taste or substitute with agave syrup or black strap molasses (use half as much). This recipe can easily be doubled.

Prep Time:	Cooking Time	Servings:
5 Mins	30 mins	3

Ingredients

- 1/2 cup quinoa.
- 1/4 teaspoon ground cinnamon.
- 1 1/2 cups almond milk.
- 1/2 cup water.
- 2 tablespoons brown sugar.
- 1 teaspoon vanilla extract (optional).
- 1 pinch salt.

Directions:

Heat a saucepan over medium heat and measure in the quinoa. Season with cinnamon and cook until toasted, stirring frequently, about 3 minutes. Pour in the almond milk, water and vanilla and stir in the brown sugar and salt. Bring to a boil, then cook over low heat until the porridge is thick and grains are tender, about 25 minutes. Add more water if needed if the liquid has dried up before it finishes cooking. Stir occasionally, especially at the end, to prevent burning.

(RECIPE - 47)

MOMMA'S POTATOES

This is a crisp, rosemary-scented alternative to fried potatoes. Dee-lish!!!

Prep Time:	Cooking Time	Servings:
15 Mins	30 mins	4

Ingredients

- 8 Yukon Gold potatoes, quartered.
- 1 tablespoon dried rosemary.
- 1/4 cup olive oil.
- salt and pepper to taste.

Directions:

01. Preheat oven to 350 degrees F (175 degrees C).

02. In a large bowl, combine the potatoes, rosemary, oil, salt and pepper. Toss well to coat.

03. Spread evenly onto cookie sheet and bake in preheated oven for 30 minutes.

(RECIPE - 48)

WHOLE WHEAT DROP BISCUITS

These are quick, easy, vegan biscuits. I especially like them with soup or vegetarian chili.

Prep Time:	Cooking Time	Servings:
5 mins	10 mins	16

Ingredients

- 1 cup whole wheat flour.
- 1 cup all-purpose flour.
- 1 tablespoon baking powder.
- 1 teaspoon salt.
- 1/4 cup canola oil.
- 3/4 cup unsweetened soy milk.

Directions:

01. Preheat the oven to 450 degrees F (220 degrees C).

02. Stir together the whole wheat flour, all-purpose flour, baking powder, and salt. Combine the oil and soy milk in a measuring cup. Pour into the dry ingredients all at once, and stir just until the dough pulls away from the sides of the bowl. Drop by heaping spoonfuls onto a baking sheet.

03. Bake for 8 to 10 minutes in the preheated oven, until the biscuits are browned on the top and bottom.

(RECIPE - 49)

CORNMEAL MUSH

This is a basic recipe for a very easy and versatile dish. You can eat it like hot cereal, or chill it and then fry it. This goes well with syrup as a breakfast dish, or with savory sauces and vegetables for dinner.

Prep Time:	Cooking Time	Servings:
5 mins	7 mins	8

Ingredients

- 1 1/4 cups cornmeal.
- 2 1/2 cups water.
- 1/2 teaspoon salt.

Directions:

01. Mix together cornmeal, water, and salt in a medium saucepan. Cook over medium heat, stirring frequently, until mixture thickens, about 5 to 7 minutes.

02. If using as cereal, spoon mush into bowls and serve with milk and sugar, if desired. If frying, pour mixture into a loaf pan and chill completely. Remove from pan, cut into slices, and fry in a small amount of oil over medium-high heat until browned on both sides. Serve with sauce of your choice.

(RECIPE - 50)

OATMEAL CHOCOLATE CHIP PANCAKES.

A tasty egg and dairy free pancake recipe! Top with organic maple syrup or ghee, or serve with warm applesauce. You can also omit the chocolate chips and add 1/4 cup hydrated raisins, 1/8 cup applesauce and cinnamon to taste.

Prep Time:	Cooking Time	Servings:
15 mins	5 mins	6

Ingredients

- 3/4 cup rolled oats.
- 3/4 cup pastry flour.
- 2 teaspoons baking powder.
- 1/2 teaspoon baking soda.
- 1/2 teaspoon sea salt.
- 1/4 cup ground flax seeds.
- 1/4 cup vegan carob chips.
- 1 1/2 cups soy milk.

Directions:

01. Preheat a lightly oiled griddle over medium heat.

02. In a medium bowl, mix rolled oats, pastry flour, baking powder, baking soda, sea salt, flax seeds, and chocolate chips. Gradually blend in soy milk.

03. Pour batter about 1/4 cup at a time onto the prepared griddle. Cook 1 to 2 minutes, until bubbly. Flip, and continue cooking until lightly browned.

(RECIPE - 51)

BLUEBERRY CORNMEAL PANCAKES

These pancakes taste really good with blueberry jam or warmed maple syrup.

Prep Time:	Cooking Time	Servings:
10 mins	15 mins	6

Ingredients

- 1 cup soy milk
- 1/2 cup water
- 1 cup whole wheat flour
- 1/2 cup stone ground cornmeal
- 1 teaspoon baking powder
- 1/2 teaspoon baking soda
- 1/4 teaspoon salt
- 1 cup fresh blueberries
- 2 tablespoons vegetable oil

Directions:

01. Preheat oven to 200 degrees F (95 degrees C).

02. In a small bowl combine the soy milk and water.

03. In a large bowl, combine the flour, cornmeal, baking powder, baking soda and salt. Stir in the soy milk mixture just until combined. Fold in the blueberries and let the batter sit for 5 minutes.

04. Lightly oil a skillet or griddle and heat over medium heat. Pour about 1/4 cup of batter onto the hot griddle and cook until pancakes are bubbly on top and edges are slightly dry looking. Turn and cook until pancakes are browned. Transfer to a baking sheet and keep warm in the oven while cooking the remaining batter. Serve warm with syrup or jam.

(RECIPE - 52)

EASY VEGAN WHOLE GRAIN PANCAKES

Delicious, easy and quick! Versatile recipe where you can use different flours and add in whatever you desire! Try using dried fruit or different types of nuts in place of the pecans.

Prep Time:	Cooking Time	Servings:
8 mins	8 mins	4

Ingredients

- 1/2 cup whole wheat flour
- 1/2 cup rye flour
- 1 tablespoon soy flour
- 1 tablespoon white sugar
- 1 1/2 teaspoons baking powder
- 1/8 teaspoon salt
- 1/8 teaspoon ground cinnamon (optional)
- 1/2 teaspoon vanilla extract (optional)
- 1/2 cup water
- 1/2 cup soy milk
- 1/4 cup chopped pecans

Directions:

01. In a medium bowl, stir together the whole wheat flour, rye flour, soy flour, sugar, baking powder, salt and cinnamon. Make a well in the center, and pour in the vanilla, water and soy milk. Mix until all of the dry ingredients have been absorbed, then stir in the pecans.

02. Heat a large skillet or griddle iron over medium heat, and coat with cooking spray. Pour about 1/3 cup of batter onto the hot surface, and spread out to 1/4 inch thickness. Cook until bubbles appear on the surface, then flip and brown on the other side. Serve warm.

(RECIPE - 53)

EGGLESS CREPES

This is a great egg-free version of the classic French crepe that can be used as as snack, lunch item, or dessert (this was developed from the vegan version).

Prep Time:	Cooking Time	Servings:
10 mins	10 mins	4

Ingredients

- 3/4 cup rolled oats
- 3/4 cup pastry flour
- 2 teaspoons baking powder
- 1/2 teaspoon baking soda
- 1/2 teaspoon sea salt
- 1/4 cup ground flax seeds
- 1/4 cup vegan carob chips
- 1 1/2 cups soy milk

Directions:

01. Preheat a lightly oiled griddle over medium heat.

02. In a medium bowl, mix rolled oats, pastry flour, baking powder, baking soda, sea salt, flax seeds, and chocolate chips. Gradually blend in soy milk.

03. Pour batter about 1/4 cup at a time onto the prepared griddle. Cook 1 to 2 minutes, until bubbly. Flip, and continue cooking until lightly browned.

(RECIPE - 54)

ULTIMATE TOFU BREAKFAST BURRITO BOWLS

Tofu scrambles up just like eggs, and with some clever spices, even non-vegans will barely notice the difference. Try setting out toppings to let family or guests assemble their own burrito bowls.

Prep Time:	Cooking Time	Servings:
15 mins	30 mins	3

Ingredients

- 4 cups self-rising flour
- 1 tablespoon white sugar
- 1 tablespoon custard powder
- 2 cups soy milk

Directions:

01. In a large bowl, stir together the flour, sugar and custard powder. Mix in the soy milk with a whisk so there are no lumps.

02. Heat a griddle over medium heat, and coat with nonstick cooking spray. Spoon batter onto the surface, and cook until bubbles begin to form on the surface. Flip with a spatula and cook on the other side until golden.

(RECIPE - 55)

WORLD'S BEST VEGAN PANCAKES

Tofu scrambles up just like eggs, and with some clever spices, even non-vegans will barely notice the difference. Try setting out toppings to let family or guests assemble their own burrito bowls.

Prep Time:	Cooking Time	Servings:
2 Mins	20 mins	4

Ingredients

- 3 tablespoons olive oil, divided
- 1 (14 ounce) package extra-firm tofu, drained
- ½ teaspoon salt
- black pepper to taste
- 1½ teaspoons onion powder
- 1½ teaspoons garlic powder
- ½ teaspoon ground turmeric
- 1 tablespoon fresh lemon juice
- 1 tablespoon olive oil
- 1 cup finely diced red onion
- 2 jalapeno peppers, seeded and chopped
- ½ teaspoon salt
- 3 cloves garlic, minced
- 2 cups chopped tomatoes
- 1½ teaspoons cumin
- ¼ cup chopped fresh cilantro
- 1 tablespoon fresh lemon juice
- 1 (15.5 ounce) can no-salt-added black beans, drained and rinsed
- 1½ cups cooked hash brown potatoes
- 1 avocado - peeled, pitted and sliced
- 1 teaspoon fresh lemon juice¼ cup chopped fresh cilantro
- 1 teaspoon hot sauce, or to taste

Directions:

01. Preheat a large, heavy skillet over medium-high heat. Add 2 tablespoons oil. Break tofu apart over skillet into bite-size pieces, sprinkle with salt and pepper, then cook, stirring frequently with a thin metal spatula, until liquid cooks out and tofu browns, about 10 minutes. (If you notice liquid collecting in pan, increase heat to evaporate water.) Be sure to get under the tofu when you stir, scraping the bottom of the pan where the good, crispy stuff is and keeping it from sticking.

02. Add onion and garlic powders, turmeric, juice, and remaining tablespoon oil and toss to coat. Cook 5 minutes more.

03. Preheat a heavy-bottomed saucepan over medium-high heat. Add oil. Cook onion and jalapenos with a pinch of salt, stirring, until translucent, about 5 minutes, Add garlic and cook, stirring, until fragrant, about 30 seconds. Add tomatoes, cumin, and remaining salt, and cook, stirring, until tomatoes become saucy, about 5 minutes. Add cilantro and lemon juice. Let cilantro wilt in. Add beans and heat through, stirring occasionally, about 2 minutes. Taste for salt and seasoning.

04. Spoon some hash browns into each bowl, followed by a scoop of beans and a scoop of scramble. Top with avocado, a squeeze of fresh lemon juice, and a sprinkle of cilantro. Serve with hot sauce.

(RECIPE - 56)

REFRESHING BANANA DRINK

This is delicious on a hot day. Also, it satisfies the thirst for a milkshake with ice cream! Using almond milk, combined with the cinnamon and banana, creates a very flavorful, sweet treat using natural flavoring.

Prep Time:	Ready Time	Servings:
10 Mins	10 mins	1

Ingredients

- 1 ripe banana.
- 3/4 cup almond milk.
- 4 ice cubes.
- 1 dash ground cinnamon.
- 1 dash vanilla extract.

Directions:

Blend banana, almond milk, ice cubes, cinnamon, and vanilla extract together in a blender on medium speed until frothy and smooth, about 1 minute.

(RECIPE - 57)

BLUEBERRY SMOOTHIE BOWL

Quick and easy blueberry smoothie topped with coconut, almonds, and banana.

Prep Time:	Ready Time	Servings:
10 Mins	10 mins	1

Ingredients

- 1 cup frozen blueberries.
- 1/2 banana.
- 2 tablespoons water.
- 1 tablespoon cashew butter.
- 1 teaspoon vanilla extract.

Toppings:
- 1/2 banana, sliced.
- 1 tablespoon sliced almonds.
- 1 tablespoon unsweetened shredded coconut.

Directions:

01. Blend blueberries, 1/2 banana, water, cashew butter, and vanilla extract together in a blender until smooth; pour into a bowl.

02. Top smoothie with sliced banana, almonds, and coconut.

(RECIPE - 58)

BERRY GOOD SMOOTHIE II

A delicious way to get your '5-a-day.' It's a quick and easy breakfast, but great any time of day! Nectarines, strawberries, and blueberries blended with nonfat milk and ice!

Prep Time:	Ready Time	Servings:
10 Mins	10 mins	2

Ingredients

- 1 nectarine, pitted.
- 3/4 cup strawberries, hulled.
- 3/4 cup blueberries, rinsed and drained.
- 1/3 cup nonfat dry milk powder.
- 1 cup crushed ice.

Directions:

In a blender combine nectarine, strawberries, blueberries, milk powder and crushed ice. Blend until smooth. pour into glasses and serve.

(RECIPE - 59)

FLAX SEED SMOOTHIE

A basic smoothie that incorporates omega 3-rich flax seed. A good source of fiber and a quick and low-calorie grab in the morning.

Prep Time:	Ready Time	Servings:
5 Mins	5 mins	1

Ingredients

- 1/2 frozen banana, peeled and cut into chunks.
- 1 cup frozen strawberries.
- 2 tablespoons flax seed meal.
- 1 cup low-fat vanilla soy milk.

Directions:

Place the banana, strawberries, flax seed meal, and soy milk into a blender. Puree until smooth.

(RECIPE - 60)

SUPER FOOD CHOCOLATE PUDDING SMOOTHIE

Feel free to make substitutions with more common ingredients (ie. regular milk for the soy or honey for the agave nectar)

Prep Time:	Ready Time	Servings:
5 Mins	5 mins	1

Ingredients

- 1 small banana, chopped
- 1/2 avocado
- 1/2 cup soy milk
- 2 tablespoons mixed frozen berries
- 2 teaspoons unsweetened cocoa powder
- 2 teaspoons agave nectar
- 1 teaspoon vanilla extract

Directions:

Blend banana, avocado, soy milk, berries, cocoa powder, agave nectar, and vanilla extract together in a blender until smooth.

(RECIPE - 61)

RAW CHIA 'PORRIDGE'

Easy, affordable raw breakfast treat. Top with your favorite fresh fruit!

Prep Time:	Ready Time	Servings:
10 mins	25 mins	1

Ingredients

- 1/4 cup chia seeds.
- 1 banana.
- 2 dates, pitted.
- 1 cup almond milk.
- 1/4 teaspoon ground cinnamon.
- salt to taste.
- 1/4 cup fresh blueberries, or more to taste.

Directions:

01. Place chia seeds in a bowl.

02. Layer banana and dates in a blender; add almond milk, cinnamon, and salt. Blend mixture until smooth and pour over chia seeds, stirring well. Let mixture sit until thickened, at least 15 minutes.

03. Stir chia 'porridge' and top with blueberries.

(RECIPE - 62)

BERRY COCONUT SMOOTHIE

Banana, berries, and almond butter are blended with coconut creating a colorful, vegan and paleo-friendly smoothie.

Prep Time:	Ready Time	Servings:
10 mins	Not Required	1

Ingredients

- 1 banana.
- ½ cup frozen blueberries.
- 1 tablespoon almond butter.
- 1 tablespoon unsweetened flaked coconut.
- ½ cup water, or as needed.

Directions:

Layer banana, blueberries, almond butter, coconut, and water in a blender; blend until smooth, adding more water for a thinner smoothie.

Cook's Note:
Any type of frozen berry can be used in place of the blueberries, if desired.

(RECIPE - 63)

FASOULIA (BREAKFAST KIDNEY BEAN DISH)

This is a traditional breakfast served in many Arabic countries. It can also be eaten for lunch or dinner in case you don't have any meat on hand, as the beans are full of protein and fiber! Very delicious! Serve and eat the traditional way, by grabbing it with pita bread

Prep Time:	Cooking Time	Servings:
15 Mins	25 mins	4

Ingredients

- 3 tablespoons olive oil
- 1 large onion, chopped
- 1 jalapeno pepper, finely chopped, or more to taste
- 1 tomato, chopped
- 2 teaspoons tomato paste
- 2 (15 ounce) cans dark red kidney beans, undrained
- 1 1/2 teaspoons ground cumin
- 1 1/2 teaspoons curry powder
- salt and black pepper to taste

Directions:

Heat olive oil in a large skillet over medium heat; cook the onion, stirring occasionally, until translucent, about 5 minutes. Stir in the jalapeno pepper; cook and stir until softened, about 5 more minutes. Mix in tomato and tomato paste; stir to combine with the onion and jalapeno pepper. Pour in the kidney beans with their liquid; stir in the cumin and curry powder. Bring the mixture to a boil, reduce heat to medium-low, and simmer until the beans are hot and the sauce has thickened, about 15 minutes.

(RECIPE - 64)

MATCHA COCONUT SMOOTHIE

Matcha green tea powder and kale make this superfood smoothie extra green. White beans add a little extra protein too!

Prep Time:	Ready Time	Servings:
10 mins	10 mins	1

Ingredients

- 1 banana
- 1 cup frozen mango chunks
- 2 leaves kale, torn into several pieces
- 3 tablespoons white beans, drained
- 2 tablespoons unsweetened shredded coconut
- 1/2 teaspoon matcha green tea powder
- 1 cup water

Directions:

Layer banana, blueberries, almond butter, coconut, and water in a blender; blend until smooth, adding more water for a thinner smoothie.

(RECIPE - 65)

AKKI ROTTI

This recipe is for Karnataka-style (Southern Indian) Akki Rotti. This savory flatbread can be enjoyed for breakfast, as a snack, or for lunch. It is very filling and contains lots of veggies to fulfill your veggie requirements for one meal in a day. Serve with the chutney or pickle of your choice.

Prep Time:	Cooking Time	Servings:
20 Mins	10 mins	4

Ingredients

- 1/2 cup green mung beans (green gram)1 cup water.
- 2 cups white rice flour.
- 1 teaspoon cumin seeds.
- 2 1/2 teaspoons finely chopped green chile peppers.
- 1/4 teaspoon asafoetida powder.
- 2 tablespoons finely chopped fresh cilantro.
- 1/2 cup unsweetened shredded coconut.
- 1/4 cup shredded carrotsalt to taste.
- 1/2 cup vegetable oil, divided.

Directions:

01. Cover the mung beans with the water and refrigerate overnight. The next day, drain the beans and reserve the soaking water.

02. In a mixing bowl, combine the mung beans, rice flour, cumin seeds, green chile, asafoetida, cilantro, coconut, shredded carrot, and salt. Gradually add the water, mixing well with your hands to form a workable dough. Use only as much water as needed (about 1/2 cup).

03. Shape the dough into balls about the size of a tennis ball. Set aside. Flatten one portion of dough into a thin round.

04. Heat 2 tablespoons of vegetable oil in a griddle or skillet over medium heat. Place the rotti in the oil, and fry until golden brown, about 30 to 40 seconds. Flip the rotti over and fry until golden. Repeat with the remaining dough, adding 2 tablespoons of oil to the griddle for each rotti. Serve hot.

Cook's Note:
When cooking the rotti, allow the griddle to cool down slightly before cooking the next one. You can also use two skillets, alternating between the two.

(RECIPE - 66)

ANNA'S SCRAMBLED TOFU

We are representing now this delicious, nutritious, and high-protein meal. Try different ingredients to suit your taste. We enjoy this meal at breakfast, but it would be suitable for any time of day. Add spinach, mushrooms, peanuts, or cashews as a topping. Serve over noodles or rice. Use additional nutritional yeast to thicken the sauce or add water to thin it.

Prep Time:	Cooking Time	Servings:
10 mins	15 mins	4

Ingredients

- 1 tablespoon olive oil, or as needed
- 1 onion, chopped
- 1 (12 ounce) package extra-firm tofu, drained and cubed
- ½ (15 ounce) can black olives, drained and halved
- 3 cloves garlic, minced
- 3 tablespoons nutritional yeast
- 1 tablespoon tamari (dark soy sauce)

Directions:

Heat olive oil in a cast iron skillet over medium heat; cook and stir onion until softened, 5 to 10 minutes. Add tofu, olives, and garlic. Cover skillet and cook, stirring occasionally, until tofu is lightly browned, about 8 minutes. Add nutritional yeast and tamari; stir until coated and nutritional yeast is dissolved, 1 to 2 minutes.

(RECIPE - 67)

FLUFFY VEGAN PANCAKES

These vegan pancakes are much fluffier than any other recipe I've had. They are also very moist and delicious! My omnivore husband loves these!

Prep Time:	Cooking Time	Servings:
10 Mins	15 mins	4

Ingredients

- 1 1/4 cups all-purpose flour
- 1 tablespoon baking powder
- 1/2 teaspoon fine sea salt
- 1/4 cup pureed extra-firm tofu
- 1 cup soy milk
- 1 tablespoon canola oil
- 1/2 cup water

Directions:

01. Whisk together the flour, baking powder, and sea salt; set aside.

02. Whisk together the tofu, soy milk, canola oil, and water. Gradually whisk the flour mixture into the tofu mixture, making sure to beat out all lumps between additions.

03. Heat a lightly oiled griddle over medium-high heat. Drop batter by large spoonfuls onto the griddle, and cook until lightly browned on the bottom. Flip, and cook until lightly browned on the other side. Repeat with remaining batter.

(RECIPE - 68)

SUNFLOWER BANANA OATMEAL

Here is a quick and delicious breakfast that can be enjoyed within minutes. Eating clean never tasted so good! Feel free to add fresh berries to give the dish a little more pizzazz.

Prep Time:	Cooking Time	Servings:
5 Mins	5 mins	3

Ingredients

- 1 3/4 cups water
- 1/4 teaspoon Himalayan pink salt
- 1 cup rolled oats
- 3 large ripe bananas, mashed
- 3 tablespoons sunflower seed butter
- 2 tablespoons agave nectar

Directions:

Bring water and salt to a boil in a saucepan; add oats and simmer until desired consistency is reached, about 5 minutes. Remove saucepan from heat and stir in bananas, sunflower seed butter, and agave nectar.

(RECIPE - 69)

ORANGE JUICE GOJI BERRIES SMOOTHIE

Orange juice with the right twist.

Prep Time:	Ready Time	Servings:
5 Mins	5 mins	1

Ingredients

- 1 cup freshly squeezed orange juice
- 1 tablespoon goji berries
- 2 slices fresh ginger

Directions:

Blend orange juice, goji berries, and ginger together in a high-powered blender until smooth and goji berries are pureed.

(RECIPE - 70)

STRAWBERRY BANANA BREEZE SMOOTHIE

Pineapple adds a bit of tropical flavor to this classic strawberry banana smoothie. Use frozen fruit for a frostier smoothie.

Prep Time:	Ready Time:	Servings:
5 mins	5 mins	2

Ingredients

- 1 medium banana
- 1 1/2 cups fresh strawberries
- 1 cup Almond Breeze Original or Unsweetened Original almondmilk
- 1/2 cup fresh or juice packed pineapple
- 1 tablespoon slivered or sliced almonds (optional)
- 1 teaspoon flax seeds (optional)

Directions:

Puree all ingredients in a blender until smooth.

Cook's Note:
Feel free to substitute chia seeds for the flax. Both sliced and slivered almonds will work.

(RECIPE - 71)

STRAWBERRY-BANANA FREEZER OATMEAL

In a hurry and don't have time to make breakfast? This recipe is ideal for a quick yet yummy breakfast. Just pop in the microwave and voila, your oatmeal is ready. Meal prep at its best.

Prep Time:	Cooking Time	Servings:
10 mins	5 mins	18

Ingredients

- 1 cup white sugar, divided.
- 2 cups fresh strawberries, sliced.
- 3 cups water.
- 2 cups almond milk.
- 2 1/2 cups old-fashioned oats.
- 1 1/2 cups bananas, mashed.
- 1 teaspoon cinnamon.
- 1 teaspoon vanilla extract.
- 1/4 teaspoon salt.
- 1/8 teaspoon ground nutmeg.
- 1/2 cup pecans, chopped.

Directions:

01. Sprinkle 1/2 cup sugar over sliced strawberries in a bowl. Let rest until juices have been released, 10 to 15 minutes.

02. Boil water and almond milk together in a large pot. Add oats and cook over medium-low heat for 5 minutes, stirring frequently. Stir in strawberries, remaining 1/2 cup sugar, bananas, cinnamon, vanilla extract, salt, and nutmeg and remove from heat. Stir in pecans.

03. Grease 18 muffin cups and fill each to the top with oat mixture, mounding a bit. Freeze 8 hours to overnight. Remove oatmeal from muffin cups and place in freezer bags or a freezer-safe container.

04. Prepare 1 frozen oatmeal cup by placing in a microwave-safe bowl and heating in a microwave oven for 1 1/2 to 2 minutes.

Cook's Note:
For thinner oatmeal, add milk. You can use any animal- or plant-based milk you like. You can slice the bananas instead of mashing, too.

(RECIPE - 72)

ORANGE PANCAKES

Oh the things I was out of when I created this dish: no milk and no eggs, but we wanted pancakes, dangit! I used flax meal to make up for the protein in the egg (a vegan trick) and substituted orange juice for milk. The result was pancakes bursting with citrus flavor. It's a new favorite in our house! Serve with butter and/or maple syrup.

Prep Time:	Cooking Time	Servings:
10 Mins	10 mins	4

Ingredients

- 2 cups white whole wheat flour
- 2 tablespoons baking powder
- 2 tablespoons ground flax meal
- 17 fluid ounces orange juice
- 1 teaspoon orange extract

Directions:

01. Whisk flour, baking powder, and flax meal together in a bowl; stir orange juice and orange extract into flour mixture until batter is well-combined.

02. Heat a lightly oiled griddle over medium-high heat, or an electric griddle to 375 degrees F (190 degrees C). Drop batter by large spoonfuls onto the griddle and cook until bubbles form and the edges are dry, 3 to 4 minutes. Flip and cook until browned on the other side, 2 to 3 minutes. Repeat with remaining batter.

(RECIPE - 73)

GREEN SMOOTHIE BOWL

Smoothie in a bowl, perfect for a quick and healthy breakfast.

Prep Time:	Ready Time	Servings:
10 Mins	10 mins	2

Ingredients

Smoothie:
- 3 cups fresh spinach.
- 1 banana.
- 1/2 (14 ounce) can coconut milk.
- 1/2 cup frozen mango chunks.
- 1/2 cup coconut water.

Toppings:
- 1/3 cup fresh raspberries.
- 1/4 cup fresh blueberries
- 2 tablespoons granola.
- 1 tablespoon coconut flakes.
- 1/4 teaspoon sliced almonds.
- 1/4 teaspoon chia seeds (optional).

Directions:

Blend spinach, banana, coconut milk, mango, and coconut water in a blender until smooth. Pour smoothie into a bowl and top with raspberries, blueberries, granola, coconut flakes, almonds, and chia seeds.

(RECIPE - 74)

VEGAN SMOOTHIE BOWL WITH CARROT AND BANANA

Looking for a healthy, yummy breakfast to start your day? Try this vegan smoothie bowl with carrots, banana, coconut, and goji berries. We used unsweetened vanilla almond milk but you can substitute with any non-dairy milk. If you like it sweeter, use some agave syrup (but we don't think it needs any extra sugar).

Prep Time:	Ready Time	Servings:
15 Mins	20 mins	1

Ingredients

- 2 pitted Medjool dates.
- 1 frozen banana, chopped.
- 1 cup coarsely chopped carrot.
- 1/2 cup unsweetened vanilla-flavored almond milk, or more to taste.
- 1/2 teaspoon ground cinnamon.
- 1/4 teaspoon ground ginger.

Toppings:

- 2 tablespoons flaked coconut.
- 1 tablespoon goji berries.

Directions:

01. Place dates in a small bowl and cover with cold water; let soak, about 5 minutes. Drain and chop.

02. Place chopped dates, banana, carrot, almond milk, cinnamon, and ginger in a blender; puree until smoothie is thick and smooth. Pour into a serving bowl.

03. Top smoothie bowl with flaked coconut and goji berries.

(RECIPE - 75)

CHIA GINGER SMOOTHIE

Cucumber, chia, ginger, and banana come together in this refreshing green smoothie that is quick and easy to prepare.

Prep Time:	Ready Time	Servings:
10 Mins	10 mins	1

Ingredients

- 1/4 cucumber, roughly chopped.
- 1 frozen banana, chopped.
- 1 teaspoon grated fresh ginger.
- 1 teaspoon chia seeds.
- 1/2 cup orange juice.
- water as needed.

Directions:

Layer cucumber, banana, ginger, and chia seeds in a blender; add orange juice. Blend mixture until smooth, adding water for a thinner smoothie.

(RECIPE - 76)

ORANGE CHIA SMOOTHIE

Oranges, mangoes, and chia seeds come together in this bright orange smoothie that is perfect for a pre- or post-workout drink.

Prep Time:	Ready Time	Servings:
10 Mins	10 mins	1

Ingredients

- 1 small orange, peeled.
- 1/2 cup frozen mango chunks.
- 1 tablespoon cashew butter.
- 1 tablespoon unsweetened coconut flakes.
- 1 teaspoon chia seeds.
- 1 teaspoon ground flax seeds.
- 1/2 cup orange juice.
- water as needed (optional).

Directions:

Layer orange, mango, cashew butter, coconut, chia seeds, and flax into a blender; add orange juice. Cover and blend mixture until smooth, adding water for a thinner smoothie.

(RECIPE - 77)

BANANA CHOCOLATE ALMOND MILK SMOOTHIE

Lactose-free and very filling, perfect for a healthy start to any morning. Add whey protein mix to add an extra long-lasting energy boost. Start the night before for fresh homemade almond milk or pick up a carton at your local grocery store to save time

Prep Time:	Ready Time	Servings:
10 Mins	10 mins	1

Ingredients

- 1 cup almond milk
- 1 banana
- 1 1/2 ounces dark chocolate bar (such as Hershey's(R) Special Dark), broken into pieces
- 1 scoop whey protein powder (optional)

Directions:

Combine almond milk, banana, dark chocolate, and protein powder in a blender; blend until smooth.

Cook's Note:
To make homemade almond milk: Soak 1 cup raw almonds in a bowl with 2 cups water, 8 hours to overnight. Transfer almonds and water to a blender and blend until it reaches a pasty consistency. Pour mixture through a cheesecloth-lined strainer into a bowl, squeezing excess liquid out of the almond meal. The remaining almond meal can be used in baking after it has been dried out a bit.

If making homemade almond milk, total time increases to about 10 hours to allow almonds to soak completely, so start the night before.

(RECIPE - 78)

ACAI SMOOTHIE BOWL

This is my favorite açaí bowl recipe, which uses very few ingredients. Acai bowls make a great breakfast and giving you two of your five a day.

Prep Time:	Ready Time	Servings:
10 Mins	10 mins	1

Ingredients

- 1 large banana, divided
- 3 1/2 ounces acai berry pulp, frozen, unsweetened
- 2 tablespoons soy milk, or more as needed
- 2 tablespoons granola

Directions:

01. Combine acai pulp, 2/3 of the banana, and 2 tablespoons of soy milk in a blender; blend until smooth, but still thick. Add more soy milk as needed; smoothie should have the consistency of frozen yogurt.

02. Slice the remaining banana. Pour thick smoothie into a bowl and top with granola and sliced bananas.

(RECIPE - 79)

RAW MANGO MONSTER SMOOTHIE

The raw adventure continues this morning with my satisfying Mango Monster Smoothie. Why is it a monster smoothie you ask? It's green, that's why...and green makes me think of monsters. This smoothie is so yummy and you can feel great drinking it because of how good it is for you!

Prep Time:	Ready Time	Servings:
10 Mins	10 mins	1

Ingredients

- 1 tablespoon flax seeds
- 2 tablespoons pepitas (raw pumpkin seeds)
- 1 ripe mango, cubed
- 1 frozen banana, quartered
- 1/3 cup water, or more to taste
- 3 ice cubes
- 2 leaves kale, or more to taste

Directions:

01. Blend flax seeds in a blender until finely ground; add pepitas and blend until ground, about 1 minute.

02. Place mango, banana, water, ice cubes, and kale in the blender; blend until smooth, kale is fully incorporated, and the smoothie is uniform in color, about 3 minutes. Thin with more water to reach desired consistency.

Cook's Note:
Freeze the banana the night before you want to make this smoothie.

(RECIPE - 80)

VEGAN MORNING SMOOTHIE

A great breakfast smoothie to pair with some toast and coffee

Prep Time:	Ready Time	Servings:
10 Mins	10 mins	1

Ingredients

- 1 banana.
- 1/3 cup frozen chopped spinach.
- 1/2 cup frozen mixed fruit.
- 1 tablespoon flax seed meal.
- 1/2 scoop vegan protein powder.
- 1 tablespoon chia seeds.
- 1/2 teaspoon matcha green tea powder.
- water to cover.

Directions:

Layer banana, spinach, mixed fruit, flax meal, protein powder, chia seeds, and matcha powder in a blender in the order listed; add enough water to cover. Cover blender and blend until smooth.

(RECIPE - 81)

PINA COLADA SMOOTHIE (VEGAN)

Very healthy breakfast or anytime meal full of protein and fiber! Enjoy!

Prep Time:	Ready Time	Servings:
10 Mins	10 mins	1

Ingredients

- 3 cubes ice cubes, or as needed.
- 1 banana.
- 1 cup fresh pineapple chunks.
- 1/2 cup coconut milk.
- 1/2 cup soy milk.
- 1 tablespoon agave nectar.
- 1 tablespoon ground flax seed.
- 1 teaspoon pure vanilla extract.

Directions:

Blend ice, banana, pineapple, coconut milk, soy milk, agave nectar, flax seed, and vanilla extract in a blender until smooth. Pour smoothie into a tall glass.

(RECIPE - 82)

ZUCCHINI SMOOTHIE

Zucchini blended with orange juice and banana makes a healthier and great-tasting breakfast smoothie. And don't worry, you can't even taste the zucchini in it.

Prep Time:	Ready Time	Servings:
5 mins	5 mins	1

Ingredients

- 1/2 cup ice cubes, or as needed (optional).
- 1/2 zucchini, shredded.
- 1/2 frozen banana.
- 1/2 cup orange juice.

Directions:

Combine ice cubes, zucchini, banana, and orange juice in a blender. Blend until smooth.

Cook's Note:
Using overripe or dark green zucchini will make this smoothie not so yummy. You can add sugar or other sweetener if you have a sweet tooth, but I find it plenty sweet from the banana.

(RECIPE - 83)

FLUFFY VEGAN PUMPKIN PANCAKES

Pumpkin puree turns these vegan pancakes orange and adds flavor. Use whatever nondairy milk you prefer. Enjoy with toppings such as nuts or bananas and syrup!

Prep Time:	Ready Time	Servings:
10 mins	10 mins	3

Ingredients

- 1 1/4 cups all-purpose flour.
- 2 teaspoons baking powder.
- 1 teaspoon pumpkin pie spice.
- 1/2 teaspoon salt.
- 1 cup soy milk.
- 1 tablespoon brown sugar.
- 3 tablespoons pumpkin puree.
- 1 teaspoon vanilla extract.
- 1 1/2 teaspoons vegetable oil.
- 1/3 cup water.

Directions:

01. Combine flour, baking powder, pumpkin pie spice, and salt in a bowl.

02. Stir milk, brown sugar, pumpkin puree, vanilla extract, oil, and water together in a second bowl; mix thoroughly. Make a well in the flour mixture, add milk mixture, and mix until evenly combined.

03. Heat a nonstick skillet over medium-high heat. Drop 1/4 cup pancake batter onto the hot skillet and cook until bubbles form and edges are dry, 3 to 5 minutes. Flip and cook until browned on the other side, 3 to 5 minutes. Repeat with remaining batter.

(RECIPE - 84)

OATMEAL-BANANA PANCAKES

These delicate, crepe-like pancakes are dairy free and easy to make. Your kids will love them! Serve with sliced bananas, syrup, and butter.

Prep Time:	Ready Time	Servings:
5 mins	10 mins	2

Ingredients

- 1/2 cup old-fashioned oatmeal.
- 3/4 cup almond milk.
- 1/2 cup almond flour.
- 1 ripe banana.
- 2 tablespoons white sugar.
- 1 teaspoon vanilla extract.
- 1/2 teaspoon ground cinnamon.
- 1/2 teaspoon baking powder.
- 1/4 teaspoon salt.
- cooking spray.

Directions:

01. Place oats in a blender and blend into a fine powder. Add almond milk, almond flour, banana, sugar, vanilla extract, cinnamon, baking powder, and salt; blend until well mixed. Let batter sit until thickened, about 10 minutes.

02. Heat a skillet over medium-high heat and coat with cooking spray. Drop 1/4 cup batter onto the hot skillet and cook until bubbles form and edges are dry, 3 to 4 minutes. Flip and cook until browned on the other side, 2 to 3 minutes. Repeat with remaining batter.

(RECIPE - 85)

APPLE-ROSEMARY STEEL-CUT OATS (INSTANT POT)

Get ready to shake up your old morning routine with an exciting new flavor of oatmeal. The woodsy taste of rosemary goes so well with the autumn flavors of cinnamon and apple in this steel-cut oatmeal done in minutes! Dried dates give it just enough sweetness, and I loved it with pecans on top.

Prep Time:	Cooking Time	Servings:
10 mins	15 mins	4

Ingredients

- 1 cup steel-cut oats.
- 2 cups water.
- 1 cup unsweetened almond milk.
- 1 large apple - peeled, cored, and diced.
- 1/3 cup dried pitted dates, diced.
- 2 teaspoons finely chopped fresh rosemary.
- 1 teaspoon vanilla extract.
- 1/2 teaspoon ground cinnamon.
- 1 pinch salt.
- 1 teaspoon chopped pecans, or to taste (optional).

Directions:

01. Place oats into a multi-functional pressure cooker (such as Instant Pot(R)). Add water, almond milk, apple, dates, rosemary, vanilla extract, cinnamon, and salt. Stir until ingredients are just combined. Close and lock the lid. Select high pressure according to manufacturer's instructions; set timer for 4 minutes. Allow 10 to 15 minutes for pressure to build.

02. Let sit for 5 minutes before releasing pressure using the quick-release method according to manufacturer's instructions, about 5 minutes. Unlock and remove the lid.

03. Stir cooked oatmeal and top with chopped pecans.

(RECIPE - 86)

BLUEBERRY MINT SMOOTHIE

Vegan, gluten-free, and nut-free!

Prep Time:	Ready Time	Servings:
10 mins	10 mins	2

Ingredients

- 2 cups frozen blueberries.
- 1 cup water.
- 1 cup fresh mint leaves.
- 1 avocado, peeled and pitted.
- 1/2 cup orange juice.
- 2 teaspoons lemon juice.

Directions:

Blend blueberries, water, mint leaves, avocado, orange juice, and lemon juice in a blender until smooth.

(RECIPE - 87)

VEGAN CHOCOLATE HEMP HIGH FIBER SMOOTHIE

This recipe is one more lovely for you because it is sweet and delicious and doesn't have any chemicals or added sugars. We make sure they are all single-ingredient options. For example, the coconut water is only coconut water, the hemp protein powder only contains hemp. You could probably use less banana and maybe peanut butter to lower the sugar and increase the protein.

Prep Time:	Ready Time	Servings:
10 mins	10 mins	1

Ingredients

- 8 fluid ounces coconut water.
- 1 sliced frozen banana.
- 1/2 cup ice cubes, or as desired.
- 3 tablespoons hemp protein powder.
- 1 tablespoon cocoa powder.

Directions:

Blend coconut water, banana, ice, hemp protein powder, and cocoa powder together in a blender until smooth.

(RECIPE - 88)

VEGAN WHOLE WHEAT APPLE PANCAKES

We're not vegan, but we love to make vegan pancakes because it cuts down on calories, fat, and unnecessary chemicals.

Prep Time:	Cooking Time	Servings:
10 mins	5 mins	4

Ingredients

- 2 cups whole wheat flour.
- 2 apples, peeled and cored.
- 1 1/2 cups almond milk.
- 1/2 cup coconut oil, melted.
- 1/4 cup water.
- 2 tablespoons baking powder.
- 2 tablespoons cane sugar, or to taste.
- 1 teaspoon ground nutmeg.
- 1/2 teaspoon ground cinnamon.

Directions:

01. Blend flour, apples, almond milk, coconut oil, water, baking powder, cane sugar, nutmeg, and cinnamon in a blender until smooth.

02. Heat a non-stick griddle over medium-high heat. Drop batter by large spoonfuls onto the griddle and cook until bubbles form and the edges are dry, 3 to 4 minutes. Flip and cook until browned on the other side, 2 to 3 minutes. Repeat with remaining batter.

(RECIPE - 89)

OATMEAL CHIA HEMP CHOCOLATE CHIP VEGAN BARS

While trying to eat healthy, I kept stuffing my face with my children's over-processed store-bought granola bars as they were around and so yummy. I came up with these as a way to save my waistline and get some 'healthy' super foods into myself and my kids....they turned out great. My 4-year-old son loves these.

Prep Time:	Cooking Time	Servings:
15 mins	15 mins	10

Ingredients

- 1/3 cup boiling water.
- 2 tablespoons ground flax seed.
- 3 cups quick-cooking oats.
- 1/4 cup chia seeds.
- 2 tablespoons hemp seed hearts.
- 1/2 teaspoon baking powder.
- 1/2 teaspoon baking soda.
- 1/4 teaspoon salt.
- 1/2 cup agave nectar.
- 1/3 cup melted coconut oil.
- 1/2 cup semisweet chocolate chips.

Directions:

01. Preheat oven to 350 degrees F (175 degrees C).

02. Mix boiling water and flax seed meal together in a bowl; set aside to thicken.

03. Combine oats, chia seeds, hemp hearts, baking powder, baking soda, and salt together in a large bowl; stir in agave nectar, coconut oil, and flax mixture until well mixed. Fold chocolate chips into mixture; press into a 9x11-inch baking pan.

04. Bake in the preheated oven until cooked through, about 15 minutes. Cool to room temperature and slice into bars. Refrigerate before removing from pan.

(RECIPE - 90)

KALE AVOCADO SMOOTHIE

This on-the-go, kale and avocado green smoothie with banana and white beans is a hearty way to start the day.

Prep Time:	Ready Time	Servings:
10 mins	10 mins	1

Ingredients

- 1/2 avocado.
- 1/2 cup frozen mango chunks.
- 1 leaf kale.
- 1/2 banana.
- 2 tablespoons drained canned white beans.
- 1/2 cup water, or more as needed.

Directions:

Layer avocado, mango, kale, banana, white beans, and water in a blender; blend until smooth, adding more water for a thinner smoothie.

(RECIPE - 91)

HEARTY PUMPKIN SPICE OATMEAL

Delicious breakfast for fall.

Prep Time:	Cooking Time	Servings:
5 mins	13 mins	2

Ingredients

- 2 cups unsweetened almond milk.
- 1/2 cup pumpkin puree.
- 2 tablespoons maple syrup.
- 1 teaspoon vanilla extract.
- 1/4 teaspoon ground cinnamon.
- 1/4 teaspoon ground nutmeg.
- 1/4 teaspoon ground cloves.
- 1 cup old-fashioned oats.

Directions:

Combine almond milk, pumpkin puree, maple syrup, vanilla extract, cinnamon, nutmeg, and cloves in a saucepan over medium heat; bring to a boil. Add oatmeal and cook, stirring frequently, until chewy and tender, 8 to 10 minutes.

Cook's Note:
Instead of using 2 cups of almond milk, you can use 1 cup milk and 1 cup water.

(RECIPE - 92)

HEARTY MULTIGRAIN SEEDED BREAD

This is a very nice, light textured multigrain bread that uses many different grains and seeds and very easy to make if you have a food processor.

Prep Time:	Cooking Time	Servings:
20 mins	30 mins	12

Ingredients

- 1 cup warm water.
- 1/4 cup white sugar.
- 1 (.25 ounce) package active dry yeast.
- 2 cups bread flour.
- 1 cup whole wheat flour.
- 1/4 cup coconut oil.
- 1 teaspoon salt.
- 1 tablespoon chia seeds.
- 1 tablespoon wheat germ.
- 1 tablespoon flax seeds.
- 1 tablespoon millet.
- 2 tablespoons hulled hemp seeds, divided.
- 2 tablespoons salted roasted sunflower seeds, divided.
- 2 tablespoons old-fashioned oats, divided.

Directions:

01. Mix warm water and sugar together in a bowl until sugar is dissolved; stir in yeast. Set aside until a creamy foam starts to form, about 5 minutes.

02. Combine bread flour, whole wheat flour, coconut oil, and salt in a food processor; pulse 4 times. Add chia seeds, wheat germ, flax seeds, millet, 1 tablespoon hemp seeds, 1 tablespoon sunflower seeds, and 1 tablespoon oats; pulse until incorporated.

03. Pour yeast mixture over flour mixture in the food processor; process until a dough ball forms, about 1 minute.

04. Turn dough into a well-oiled large bowl and cover with a damp towel; allow to rise in a warm area until doubled in size, about 1 hour.

05. Punch dough down and knead a few times. Form dough into an oblong shape and place in a greased bread pan. Lightly press the remaining hemp seeds, sunflower seeds, and oats onto the loaf. Cover with a damp towel and let rise in a warm area for 30 minutes.

06. Preheat oven to 350 degrees F (175 degrees C).

07. Bake in the preheated oven until cooked through and crust is lightly browned, about 30 minutes. Cool bread in the pan for 5 minutes before transferring to a wire rack to cool completely.

(RECIPE - 93)

AVOCADO SMOOTHIE

Do not let the ingredients scare you! This antioxidant-rich smoothie will brighten your skin, fill you up, and taste like the most delicious smoothie you've ever had! Add additional milk if desired.

Prep Time:	Ready Time	Servings:
5 mins	5 mins	1

Ingredients

- 12 fluid ounces unsweetened almond milk.
- 1 avocado, peeled and pitted.
- 1 tablespoon honey

Directions:

Combine almond milk, avocado, and honey in a blender; blend until smooth.

Cook's Note:
Feel free to substitute almond milk for skim milk, coconut milk, or flaxseed milk!

(RECIPE - 94)

DETOX SMOOTHIE

This green goodness is something I threw together this morning! So good!

Prep Time:	Ready Time	Servings:
5 mins	5 mins	1

Ingredients

- 1 Granny Smith apple.
- 1 1/2 cups fresh spinach.
- 1 cup blueberries.
- 1/2 cup soy milk.
- 4 ice cubes (optional).

Directions:

Combine Granny Smith apple, spinach, blueberries, soy milk, and ice cubes in a blender; blend until smooth.

CHIA PINEAPPLE SMOOTHIE

This chia and pineapple smoothie is a refreshing and filling way to start the day!

Prep Time:	Ready Time	Servings:
10 mins	10 mins	2

Ingredients

- 2 bananas.
- 1 cup frozen pineapple.
- 2 tablespoons almond butter.
- 1 tablespoon chia seeds.
- 1 cup water.

Directions:

Combine bananas, pineapple, almond butter, and chia seeds in a blender; add water. Blend until smooth.

(RECIPE - 96)

CUCUMBER PEAR SMOOTHIE

Cucumber, pineapple, and pear are blended with ginger and a secret ingredient (white beans!) creating a refreshing on-the-go smoothie.

Prep Time:	Ready Time	Servings:
10 mins	10 mins	1

Ingredients

- 1/4 cucumber, chopped.
- 1 pear, chopped.
- 1/4 cup frozen pineapple.
- 2 tablespoons drained canned white beans.
- 1 tablespoon chopped fresh parsley.
- 1/2 teaspoon grated fresh ginger.
- 1/2 cup water, or as desired.

Directions:

Layer cucumber, pear, pineapple, white beans, parsley, and ginger in a blender; add water. Cover and blend mixture until smooth, adding more water for a thinner smoothie.

(RECIPE - 97)

SMOOTHIE BOWL WITH MANGO AND COCONUT

A yummy vegan smoothie with mango, coconut, and vanilla.

Prep Time:	Ready Time	Servings:
10 mins	10 mins	1

Ingredients

- 1 1/2 cups frozen mango chunks.
- 1 cup vanilla-flavored almond milk.
- 1 frozen banana, chopped.
- 1 tablespoon unsweetened coconut cream.
- 1/4 teaspoon vanilla extract.
- 1 tablespoon flaked coconut.
- 1 teaspoon goji berries.
- 1/2 teaspoon chia seeds.

Directions:

01. Place mango chunks, almond milk, banana, coconut cream, and vanilla extract in a blender; puree until smoothie is thick and smooth. Pour into a serving bowl.

02. Top smoothie bowl with flaked coconut, goji berries, and chia seeds.

Cook's Note:
You can use any vanilla-flavored milk. Use less milk if you prefer a thicker smoothie. I happened to have an open can of coconut cream in the fridge and felt it needed extra coconut but you can omit that if you like.

(RECIPE - 98)

DREAMY CASHEW BUTTER SMOOTHIE WITH BANANA, BERRY, DATES, AND FLAX

It is a Wake Up breakfast, Without Coffee Smoothie! Yummy and healthy - try it out.

Prep Time:	Ready Time	Servings:
5 mins	5 mins	1

Ingredients

- 1 ripe banana.
- 1/2 cup cold unsweetened almond milk.
- 1/3 cup frozen blueberries.
- 2 dates, pitted and chopped, or more taste.
- 1 1/2 tablespoons flax seeds.
- 1 tablespoon cashew butter, or more to taste.

Directions:

Blend banana, almond milk, blueberries, dates, flax seeds, and cashew butter together in a blender on high speed until smooth.

(RECIPE - 99)

LIGHT AND FLUFFY VEGAN WAFFLES

Simple, vegan waffle recipe for a lazy weekend morning. Cooked waffles store well in the fridge or frozen and reheat in the toaster, if allowed to cool fully and kept separated between sheets of parchment paper.

Prep Time:	Cooking Time	Servings:
10 mins	30 mins	6

Ingredients

- 1/2 cup warm water.
- 2 tablespoons flaxseed meal.
- 2 cups all-purpose flour.
- 2 tablespoons baking powder.
- 1 tablespoon white sugar.
- 1/2 teaspoon salt.
- 1 3/4 cups almond milk.
- 1/4 cup vegetable oil.
- 1/4 cup applesauce.
- 1 teaspoon vanilla extract.

Directions:

01. Combine water and flaxseed meal in a medium-sized bowl. Set aside for 5 minutes.

02. Combine flour, baking powder, sugar, and salt in a large mixing bowl. Mix well.

03. Add almond milk, oil, applesauce, and vanilla extract to flaxseed mixture. Combine until smooth. Add to flour mixture and stir until just combined.

04. Preheat a waffle iron according to manufacturer's instructions.

05. Add 1/3 cup waffle batter to the preheated waffle iron and cook until waffle is golden brown and the iron stops steaming, about 5 minutes. Repeat with remaining batter.

Cook's Note:
You can use any milk substitute that you'd like, such as soy milk.

(RECIPE - 100)

QUICK VEGAN BREAKFAST BOWL WITH FRUIT

A quick and easy vegan breakfast that is full of vitamins - I prefer to use berry-flavored soy yogurt, but any flavor will do. You can add any kind of fruit topping you like.

Prep Time:	Ready Time	Servings:
5 mins	5 mins	1

Ingredients

- 1 (6 ounce) container vegan strawberry yogurt.
- 1 teaspoon spirulina powder.
- 2 tablespoons cornflakes cereal.
- 3 fresh strawberries, halved.
- 1/2 large kiwifruit, peeled and sliced.
- 1 tablespoon fresh blueberries.
- 1 tablespoon chopped pecans.

Directions:

Combine yogurt and spirulina powder in a bowl; mix well. Top with cornflakes, strawberries, kiwifruit, blueberries, and pecans.

(RECIPE - 101)

VEGAN HAZELNUT SPREAD

A delicious spread without dairy and refined sugar - think of it as a vegan version of Nutella(R) without the use of palm oil.

Prep Time:	Ready Time	Servings:
10 mins	10 mins	20

Ingredients

- 1 cup whole raw hazelnuts.
- 1/4 cup unsweetened cocoa powder.
- 1/4 cup agave nectar.
- 1/4 cup unsweetened almond milk, or more as needed.
- 2 tablespoons melted coconut oil.
- 1 teaspoon vanilla extract.

Directions:

Combine hazelnuts, cocoa powder, agave nectar, almond milk, coconut oil, and vanilla extract in the bowl of a food processor. Pulse until smooth, adding more almond milk if mixture is too thick. Spoon into jars and store in the refrigerator for up to 2 weeks.

Made in United States
Orlando, FL
20 January 2024